Marianne E. Meyer
Cranberry Power Fruit
Handbook to the Methuselah Berry
Sensational Healing Successes &
Delicious Cranberry Recipes for the Healthy Kitchen

Produce and publishing
BoD - Books on Demand, Norderstedt
ISBN 978-3-743181595

The information introduced in this book was carefully researched and imparted in all conscience. However, author and publisher do not take any liability for damages of any nature that could emerge directly or indirectly from the usage or application of the data in this book which is for interested parties and education.

© 2017 by Marianne E. Meyer, Tavira, Portugal
All rights are with the author
drmarianneemeyer@gmail.com
www.marianne-e-meyer.com

Some other books by M. E. Meyer:

How Water Connects our Worlds
Family Code – Death is Not the End
Migrant Birds on Wheels
Spirulina für ältere Menschen
Psyllium - So bekommen Sie Ihr Fett weg
Spirulina für Kinder
Spirulina, das blaugrüne Wunder

Marianne E. Meyer
Apartado 320, P-8801 Tavira

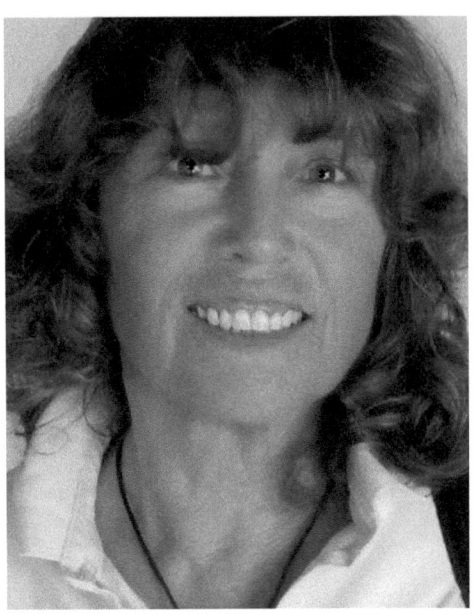

Marianne E. Meyer has already passed through many stages of life with the focus on self-help and learned: We are our own best teachers, healers, and spiritual leaders. Formerly a doctor's assistant, she later studied with a focus on family therapy and gerontology in Frankfurt. She then studied food science in the USA. The dissertation case study on immune defense and Spirulina she published in her bestseller *Spirulina, das blaugrüne Wunder*. The author lived 10 years in the US, intervening in Southern Hesse, Portugal, and Morocco. Until recently, she worked temporarily with maladjusted adolescents in Portugal. She is inspired by a pioneering spirit and a passionate dedication on the well-being of the people.

Marianne E. Meyer

CRANBERRY
POWER FRUIT

Handbook to the Methuselah Berry

Sensational Healing Successes and delicious cranberry recipes for the healthy kitchen

Layout: I would like to thank the Cranberry Marketing Committee (CMC) - Cranberries from the USA for the friendly providing of photos.

Other photo credits
Cover back and page 2: R. Taylor
Cover, typography & typesetting: M. Meyer

TABLE OF CONTENT

Preface	**10**
I. INTRODUCTION	**11**
Every second woman has a urinary tract infection	13
Candida or cystitis?	14
The anti-candida diet has many benefits	14
II. NORTH AMERICAN BERRY ON THE RISE	**15**
The French celebrate the fire-red fruit	15
Success measured at trade exhibitions	16
Product range: almost weekly new outputs	16
Fresh and frozen cranberries - keepability	17
Sirup, concentrate, and powder	17
Cranberry juices and juice mixtures	18
Cranberry dry fruits & snacks	18
Nutritional analysis of cranberry products	19
Acid fruits conquer the media	19
Superpower against bacteria.	20
III. FACTS AND FOLKLORE	**21**
The cranberry botanized	22
Habitat requirements	22
Growth process of the capricious roots	24
The Harvest of cranberry: a berry sports festival	24
Dry harvest: when berries are jumping	24
Wet harvest: swimming is cool	24
History and mystery	24
Use: a good fit with cranberries	26
Awaken cranberries the joie de vivre of the cow?	26
In comparison with the cowberry..	27
IV. HEALTH ENHANCING CONTENTS	**28**
What's in the redskin?	28
Secondary metabolites: Can we reverse the clock?	28
How do the phytochemicals work?	29
Oligomeric procyanidins (OPC) or proanthocyanidins (PAC)	29
How many antioxidants do we consume?	29
Polyphenol comparison of conventional beverages	30

Polyphenol comparison of common beverages 30
Polyphenol comparison of common foods 30
Health effects of PAC/OPC 30
Lutein and zeaxanthin prevent macular degeneration 31
Vitamin C - ascorbic acid - E 300 31
Average analysis of cranberry juice 31

IV. DISEASE PREVENTION AND CURE FROM A - Z 32

Arteriosclerosis: stretching for the veins 32
Bladder infections: Cranberries dispel Coli bacteria 33
Cancer: Special nutrients delay cancer growth 33
Candida: Cranberry helps to prevent fungi 35
Caries: The cranberry can scare away germs 36
Cataract: The OPC of the power berry protects the lens 36
Cystitis: When the bladder is plaguing 37
Diabetes: 240 ml Cranberry juice ensures constant blood glucose levels 37
Food poisoning: Cranberries protect against salmonella 39
Gastritis: Cranberry juice prevents the docking of Helicobacter pylori 39
Gingivitis: cranberries for powerful biting 40
Heart disease: red card for heart diseases 40
Immune deficiency: bathing fun without bladder problems 41
Intestinal infections: Cranberry juice prevents ulcers 42
Irritable bladder: the bladder as a mirror of the psyche 43
Kidney stones: cranberry for prevention 44
Macular degeneration: lutein and zeaxanthin guard against 44
Pancreas: when parasitic fungi are plagueing 45
Periodontitis: Cranberries prevent bacteria from adhering to teeth 45
Plaque/bleeding gums: cranberry juice for prevention 45
Poor digestion: The bitter substances of the cranberry stimulate gastric juices ... 46
Rheumatoid arthritis (RA): Can crippling form back? 46
Salmonellosis: healthy despite rotten meat 47
Stomach ulcer: Cranberry juice dispels Helicobacter 47
Stroke: Cranberry's polyphenols prevent brain attacks 47
Thrombosis: prophylaxes instead of support stockings 48
Urinary tract infections: Belly shows can end painfully 49

The miraculous transformation of rods into spheres 51
Prevention with the redskin is a necessity 51
What else can we do for the bladder? 51
Can the cranberry turn the clock back? 52

V. PROGRESS REPORTS: EXPERIENCE AND PERCEPTION 54

Distress during coitus 54
Distress after coitus 54
General resistance: the barefoot woman from Beerfelden 54
Cranberry mobilizes memory capacity 55
Painful bladder as blown away 55
Short story for the coincidence album 55
After a few days a lot of energy and super coagulation test 55
How much juice does the bladder boost? 56
If we can tolerate little acidity 56
Cranberry tip for bright minds 57

VI. REFINED RECIPES OF THE HEALTH CUISINE 58

Spicy universal mash 58
Sweet universal mash 58

Salads 60
    Asparagus salad with "ham" strips 60
    Cranberry dressing 60
    Cranberry vegetable salad 61
    Millet and cranberry salad 61
    Red, raw vegetable salad 61
    Spinach salad with cranberries 61
    Tabbouleh 61

Soups, snacks, and appetizers 62
    Acranjoli 62
    Avocado puree 63
    Carrot soup with cranberries and pita 63
    Flatbread (chapati) 63
    Green spelt soup 64
    Kichari with cranberries 65
    Naan bread 65
    Roasted and salted cranberries 65
    Sweet-and-sour cranberry coconut soup 65

Main courts without beheading 66
   Apple curd casserole with cranberries 66
   Aubergine cranberry pizza 67
   Cranberry fresh cheese balls on salad 69
   Cranberry nut bread 69
   Canneloni rolls 69
   Cranberry pumpkin risotto 69
   Fried pumpkin with dried 70
   "Meat" loaf 70
   Potato salad with cranberry, celery and walnuts 70
   Pasta with dried cranberries 71
   Pizza with dried cranberries 72
   "Rehragout" with dried cranberries and mushrooms 72
   Spaghetti "bolognese" 73
   Spicy reddish muffins 73
   "Turkey breast" with cranberry walnut chutney) 73
   Zucchini boats, loaded with tofu 74
   Zucchini pancake with apple sauce 74

Cakes, desserts & sweets 76
   Ananas (pineapple) pie on the head 76
   Cranberry almond bar 77
   Cranberry apple strudel with walnuts 77
   Cranberry chocolate delight 77
   Cranberry jelly 77
   Cranberry sauce 78
   Cranberry sorbet 78
   Cranberry walnut muffin 78
   Fruit ice cream with nut 78
   Fruity soft ice cream 78
   Papaya - pep up 78
   Chocolate cranberry walnut cake 79
   Chocolate nut fruit bars 80
   Vanilla and cranberry waffles 80

***Happy Hour*: vital food dips & spreads** 81
   Chickpea cranberry dip 81
   Herbal cranberry cream 81
   Immuno power paste 81
   Tofu deli dip 81
   Tart lemon mouse 82

Cranberry mixtures 82
    Anti-stress shake 82
    Artery power drink 82
    Cashew cranberry mix 82
    Cranberry milk 82
    Fruity cranberry fizz 82
    Nerve cooler 82
    Paradise punch 82
    Pineapple cranberry juice 83
    Pink dream 83
    Souls comforter 83
    Thanksgiving punch 83

Cocktails & Dreams 84
    Cosmopolitan 84
    Cran-Appler 84
    Cranberry Collins 84
    Sex on the Beach 84
    Save Sex on the Beach 84
    Cranberry Colada 85
    Vocal cord delight 85

Free forum for free questions 86

Acknowledgments 86

References 86

Alphabetical index 89

For your notes 97

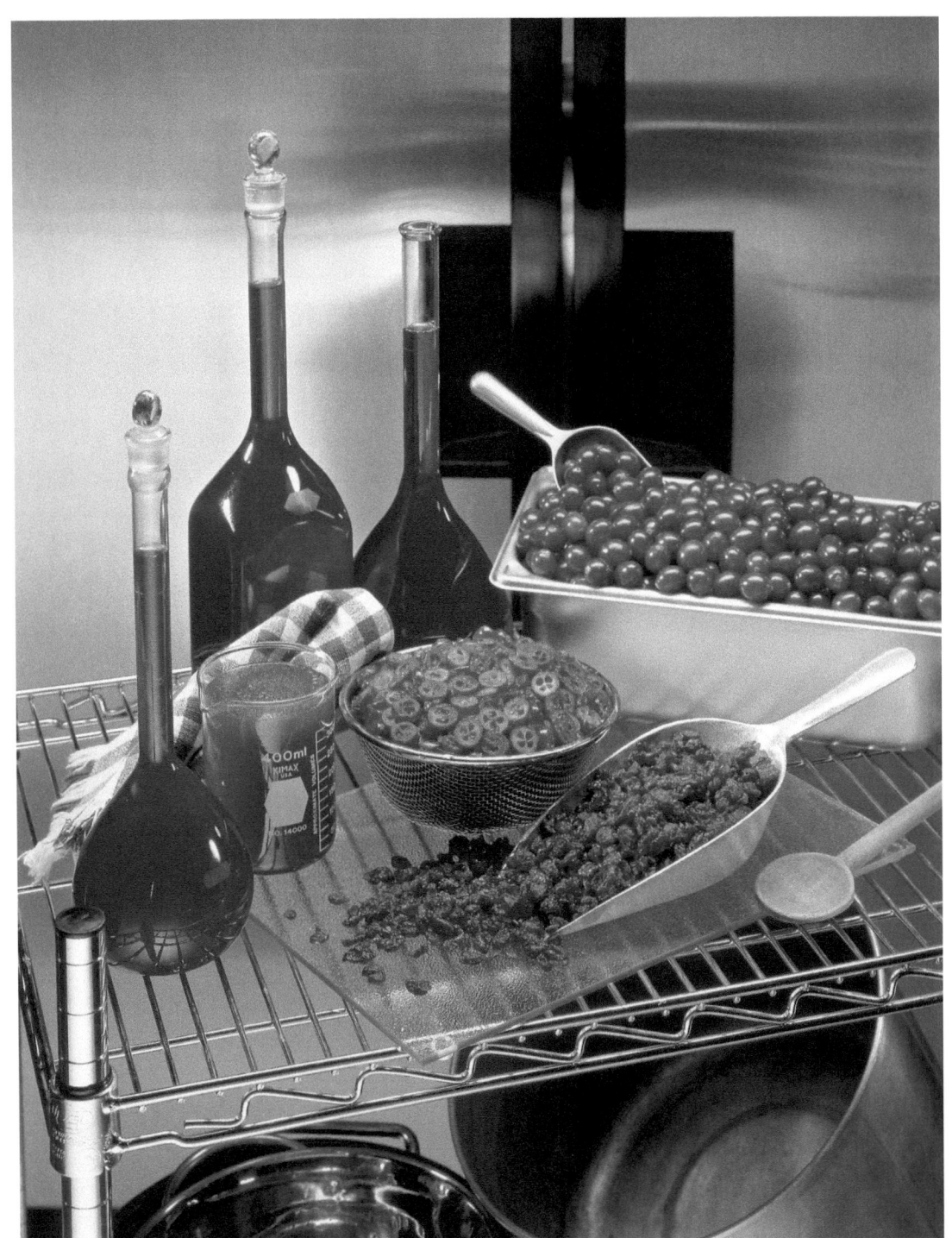

Preface

It looks as if spiritual children also choose their parents. Sometimes they even wait for many years until their parents are ready. In the mid1990s I walked with my friends from the neighborhood in the Santa Monica mountains. I asked Bette Rohm if she had heard of *speaking in tongues*. Yes why? She asked. I just realized that my mother told me that she heard women suddenly talking in a foreign language. We belonged to a splinter group of the New Apostolic Church. Bette said:

That's known in the Seventh-day Adventist Church, too. So we have a similar upbringing. Passing a ruby blooming hibiscus bush, I said: Those are edible, good for the immune system. Bette stopped abruptly. Huh? What? Um! Gazing at me, she said: You'll have a message for us in 10 or 12 years. Wide-eyed with goosebumps all over, I asked: What kind of message? Had Bette a vision? Was s h e now speaking in tongues? Um ... something with crystal ... wait ... What do you mean, Christ? Maybe. I don't know I ... cranberries? No, wait, it's got to do with water. Huh? Dunno. (Meyer 2017, p. 159)

It was true that I had written down this incident, but had long since forgotten it, when the director of the Windpferd publishing house, Mrs. Jünemann, asked me to write a book about the cranberry.

Meanwhile, the acid berries had triggered a real hype. That's why I'm all the more surprised that there is still no reference book in English.

So why me? Why was I selected to write a book about the North American Cranberry? I was born on Sunday after Thanksgiving. But that will not be the reason. Rather, that my father's grandfather had emigrated to Northern California in 1902 and I would like to find his descendants.

Since my biography consists of a collection of coincidences I might be led again. And if the cranberry book will be well received in the Anglo-American market it might be that a relative of my father will read the book about the bladder curative. For my grandmother Maria the child of love who may have driven her father into the wide world had bladder problems, so perhaps her relatives in the USA as well. To find my great-grandfather would be to prove the existence of the spiritual world and to confirm the cosmic laws. To understand this, you would need to read my book *Family Code*.

But perhaps you want to know how I came to write the cranberry book:

A Russian doctor living in Braunschweig provided the ignition spark. Alfira Weihe wrote a comment on my website on June 7, 2006. She had perceived me in the ARD *Wunschbox* with Ingo Dubinski as a committed Spirulina expert. Since then she has been consuming the blue-green algae and would like to translate my bestseller *Spirulina, das blaugrüne Wunder* into Russian.

On the same day, I called the head of the Windpferd publishing house. Monika Jünemann asked me if I wanted to write a book about the natural appetite suppressant hoodia or the cranberry. Destiny or guidance? Both topics are a big hit. Already as a 16-year-old, I'd been messing with appetite suppressants. I thought, hey, that's it. In the following week, however, I was bothered by my irritable bladder. I interpreted this in the way, as to go for the urinary tract healing berry. To follow in the steps of Dr. Ruth K. Westheimer, I'm also not a person beating around the bush and will make the taboo topic sociable again.

I. INTRODUCTION

In North America since 1621 every end of November a red carpet is laid out for a redskin that is worth its weight in gold. Whether in California, Texas or New England, Americans can barely imagine the prelude to the Christmas season without the cranberry.

When the Puritan pilgrims no longer liked in England reached the coast of Massachusset in 1620, the Indians made them acquainted with the cranberry. After the seven-week sea voyage on the Mayflower, they may have suffered from vitamin C deficiency.

The natives have valued the versatility of the fruit hundreds of years before regarding it as a symbol of peace and friendship.

Part I. shows you that you are not alone with bladder problems. And since it is hard to tell if the reason is a bacteria or a yeast, you can test it with cranberries or the anti-candida diet.

So far the cranberries in the North American cooking were only celebrated on Thanksgiving similar to the peanut. But this will probably change soon. In part II. you learn about the wide range of cranberry products and the nutritional value of the fruit.

Part III. tells you facts and folklore: how cranberries are grown and harvested and their value compare to the cowberry.

At the moment international research is running at full speed. They show: The *Vaccinium macrocarpon* is a real cornucopia of powerful antioxidants. It has caused a great stir in France: The French Ministry of Health has attributed the acidic fruit a very special healing potential: it prevents the adhesion of bacteria! So the consumption of cranberries prevents infections caused by bacteria. Therefore, I am quite confident about their glorious future: They will become a permanent ingredient of daily food preparation: at the latest when people have realized how easy they can naturally strengthen their immune system.

American researchers have found that we can even protect ourselves against the No. 1 killer: the regular consumption of cranberries slows the buildup of plaques in arteries, makes the vessels elastic again and prevents heart and circulatory diseases. You can find out which of the ailments you can get rid of by the healing powers of the allrounder, in part IV. DISEASES PREVENTION AND HEALING FROM A – Z.

Until recently the nutritious redskins were only colored blobs on the American feast days table. A turkey without cranberry sauce is unthinkable in the USA. But I would like to bet that

chefs of all countries will surpass each other in the future with cranberry creations.

Even the children do not have to do without their peanut butter & jelly sandwiches. The sweet bread spreads will get cranberries mixed into in the future: apple, apricot or orange gels will then shine in a reddish color. Also, in private kitchens, the trend berry will soon be indispensable: Fresh, frozen or dried it gives every vegetable, meat or fish dish a special touch. My readers can convince themselves of this in the extensive recipe section in Part V. REFINED RECIPES OF THE HEALTH CUISINE. It will be not possible to imagine muesli and salad without the round healthy berry anymore. We are facing a whole new era of nutrition. Health-conscious people around the world will soon learn to appreciate the healing power of the cranberry!

Every second woman has a urinary tract infection

The reason why women suffer much more frequently from urinary infections is the anatomy: the female urethra is 5-8 times shorter than the male with 2½ to 4 cm. In cases of urinary bladder or urethral infections, an increased urge to urinate may occur, often associated with burning during urination. Young women also suffer from inflammation of the urinary tract. One-third of all sufferers have recurring ailments of the lower urinary tract often associated with agitation and sexual pain. Women are also plagued by increased urge to urinate during menopause. Passing urine twice or more frequently at night is called nocturia pointing to an overactivity or dysfunction of the bladder muscle. There could also be serious physical problems, such as cardiac insufficiency or diabetes.

In conversations, it is always clear how little we know about our body. My interest in the causes of illness results from my experiences as a frequently ill child. My symptoms covered with drugs led to new suffering. It was not until much later that I learned disease is the organism's attempt to excrete toxic substances. It is essential to strengthen our body's defenses better paying for maintaining our health than for disease.

Candida or cystitis?

During my preparatory work for this book, I found the term "Candida cystitis" in the literature. I thought that must be it. Because of my antibiotics flood in childhood, I had suffered Candida infections ever since I can remember, especially in stressful situations. At school, the yeast fungi took over in class tests itching at the head, in the ears, on the body. My teacher said: Leave the little animals alone. If they had left me alone. Also later, when I was overtaxed and stressed, the parasites could always take over again. For example, I wrote three books in 1997/98 in a single year and gave my first lecture in front of alternative practitioners. At that time the parasitic yeasts increased because I ate less carefully. Normally with diet and daily immune activation with Spirulina and Colloidal Silver I always keep them in check. Why could they always take over again? I give you an example: Ten years ago, I interviewed a holistic beauty therapist specializing in anti-aging and cellulite for a book project. Since I gave her my Spirulina book, she gave me Jacky Gehring's "BodyReset" which she recommends to her overweight clientele. In this, the author offers a basic nutritional plan to reduce the acid level in the body. I also took off 2 kilos and weighed again 52: my ideal weight. I ate mainly potatoes, salad, vegetables, sweet apples and bananas and drank a glass of red wine in the evening all allowed in the book. The problem is just:

Every organism reacts differently. That is why it often takes a long time before we find the right food.

Mine reacted with itching on all warm spots. I feel best avoiding sugar, alcohol, white flour and other goodies the yeasts thrive on. So I stopped Jacky's diet and gave her publication to somebody with weight problems. In my book *Spirulina, das blaugrüne Wunder* I granted the Candida albicans ten pages.

By the way, unsweetened cranberry juice is also recommended by Dr. Allan Sachs, author of the book *The Authoritative Guide to Grapefruit Seed Extract* as an accompanying treatment for Candida infections. In vitro studies did not show any specific antifungal effects against Candida albicans. However, it proved effective against dermatophytes and other fungi. (Swartz and Medrek 1968, Cipollini and Stiles 1992). Since only a few people know which fungi they are haunted by, we better test cranberry juice and other natural remedies. Then we can be sure not to be taken in by any interest group. For the pharmaceutic and chemical industry, effective natural remedies are of no interest. Only we can benefit from it. And with our finances, it would go uphill. Prerequisite: The health insurance companies stop their money incineration plant and rely on sustainability in the health care system.

The anti-candida diet has many benefits

One is to test if you suffer from Cystitis or a yeast infection. The symptoms are similar. Frequent urination and burning sensation, just to name two. Most of us have Candida in our guts. In small colonies, they are usually harmless. But eating sweets, wheat, and starchy vegetables, drinking wine and beer, taking antibiotics and having permanent stress can lead to overgrowth.

Since Candida albicans thrives on sugar, I brought the sweet fruits to the neighbors. Eating sour apples, papaya, grapefruit, avocado and sour berries I keep the opportunistic fungus at bay. The Candida cells require sugar to build their cell walls, spread out and turn into their more virulent, fungal form (Han et al. 2011). We better avoid starchy vegetables, preferring kale, brown rice, millet, buckwheat, and quinoa.

White flour, sugar, and alcoholic beverages are taboo during the expulsion phase.

There is a lot of green stuff: dandelion, plantain, comfrey and other wild herbs, chard, green cabbage, barley grass and Spirulina. The fungi don't like these oxygen carriers. This gas, which accounts for 21% of the air kills the yeast. Between the meals, a few drops of grapefruit seed extract or colloidal silver act like a club. Probiotics such as kefir, sauerkraut or organic yogurts consumed with meals colonize the intestine with beneficial bacteria. This applies for fructooligosaccharides too. These FOS mixtures are produced commercially, based on inulin degradation or transfructosylation processes. Studies have shown that up to 20 grams per day are well tolerated (Carabin and Flamm 1999).

FOS are also found in food such as asparagus, bananas, barley, blue agave, chicory, garlic, jícama leeks, and topinambour. With this diet, the intestinal flora will be rebuilt in a few weeks. And, if the microbiome is in order again our immune system's largest organ, the intestine will keep up our well-being.

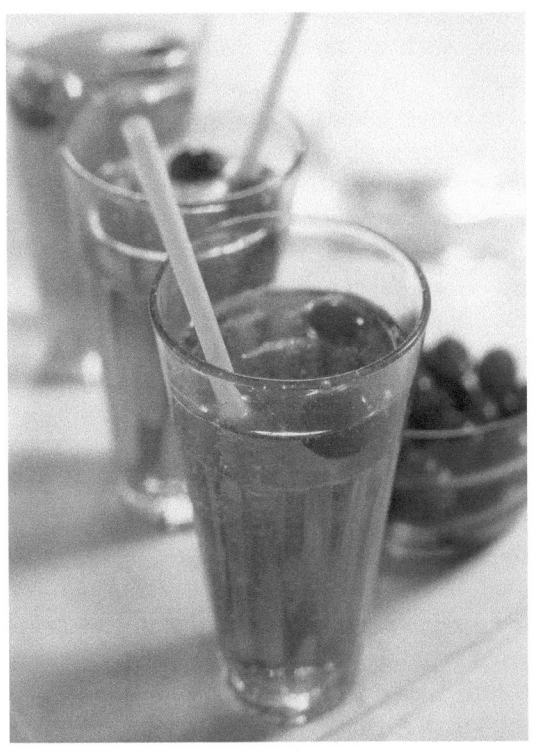

II. NORTH AMERICAN BERRY ON THE RISE

The red rounds are overrunning us. Almost every week new research results are announced testifying that cranberries and cranberry products have a positive effect on health in various ways. Compared to other fruits, cranberries contain very many antioxidative components. Antioxidants protect our cells from free radical attack. These arise as a by-product of metabolic processes or by external stress, e. g., rays, artificial substances, nicotine, and alcohol.

Native Americans may not have known the exact effects of their curative berry. However, they have already used cranberries in the past to alleviate a variety of conditions: from simple abdominal pain to pain, presumably from cancer.

Everything in America is known to be bigger, wider and higher than in the rest of the world: cars, houses, trees. Why should not the berries also have more impressive proportions? Accordingly, the Vaccinium macrocarpon grows to olive-to-cherry-sized. Their European relative less respected by research, the lingon- or cowberry (Vaccinium vitis-idaea), has only the size of a pea.

The large cranberry (Vaccinium macrocarpon) owes its name American, Canadian or arctic cranberry to the Pilgrim Fathers emigrated from England. They called the fruit craneberry because the delicate pinkish-white flowers with lateral inflorescences reminded them of the head and beak of a crane. Later the name was shortened to cranberry. Some also called them bear berries as bears were feeding on them.

Thanks to their fresh, sour taste, the red fruits gained a firm place in North American cuisine. The natives introduced the cranberry to starving English settlers in Massachusetts, who incorporated the fruit into Thanksgiving. So since the 17th century, berries are obligated with meals of the traditional feast. Certain ingredients, as well as a wax layer, are responsible for the fact that the cranberries of the later varieties are still edible in winter. Because of the particularly good storage capacity, sailors took them on their long journeys. They knew that their high vitamin C content could protect them from scurvy.

Originally cranberries were found in the raised mosses of New England. In the Northwest of the USA and in Canada, they are also cultivated and marketed extensively. In some German moors they were naturalized as neophytes, that is, brought into this region by people after the discovery of America in the late 15th century. They belong to the so-called homosporous plants, that is, they produce spores of one kind only that are not distinguished by sex. The spores of homosporous plants grow into bisexual gametophytes producing both male and female germ cells.

The cowberry flatters the palate rather than the more dominant cranberry tasting as a mixture of berries and apples. Sweetened, they have an exotic taste. Every time I test a new brand, I am amazed at the different flavor.

The French celebrate the fire-red fruit

In bars, cranberries give cocktails a certain kind of buzz. The juice of the little red fruit also conquered pharmacies and health food stores. Cranberries are on everyone's lips. The reason: their unique ingredients are chasing bacteria away. Vive la baie rouge de l'Amérique! The AFSSA (Agence Française de Sécurité Sanitaire des Aliments), the French food inspection authority, was the first in the world to approve a health certificate for cranberry juice. Since April 2004, products containing cranberries have been shown to help prevent the adhesion of Escherichia coli bacteria in the urinary tract. Masashi Matsushima and his Japanese team can verify the health claim cranberries inhibit Helicobacter pylori bacteria, which are responsible for 80% of gastric ulcers and possibly cancer (2008).

For the application for the official recognition of the health potential of cranberries, AFSSA presented a comprehensive collection of scientific studies. These affirm the role played by the berries for the health of the urinary tract. The relevance of the proanthocyanidins was pointed out. In a health-related statement on 29 January 2004, the AFSSA states that "the statement - contributes to the reduction of the attachment of different E. coli bacteria to the mucous membranes of the urinary tract - only applies to the Vaccinium macrocarpon and the powder of the fruit juice of this plant. The French Food Control Authority stated in the same opinion:

"A daily consumption of at least 36 mg proanthocyanidins" from cranberry powder has a positive effect on the health of the bladder and urinary tract ".

For about one Euro or Dollar a day we can promote our health, mainly of the bladder, intestine, stomach, heart, palate, blood, veins, and eyes. You better find out yourself in what way the American redskins can help you. Thru our experience we generate knowledge which is the true science.

Success measured at trade exhibitions

The organizers of BioFach registered a visitor record in the world event of the BioFach in February 2006: 37,426 professionals from all over the world met in Nuremberg. At the stand of a well-known supplier, the rush was heavy at the end of the fair. And this is why it happened: In the first three days, the committed naturalist had generously distributed his sachets with Urovit® cranberry powder. A few women came to the stand on the last day and ordered the microfine red granules. The striking success speaks for the rapid effect of the North American miracle showing the widespread infections of the urinary tract. I also found out that when I speak of the healing power of the cranberry with bladder problems, I have the undivided attention of the women.

In Berlin, red berries rained on the Berlin bears, in 2006. More than 80 cranberry products filled the shelves at the Fruit Logistica in Germany's federal capital. The international fruit trade is booming: 35,635 visitors, 22% more than in 2005. At the US pavilion, the guests saw red. They tasted various varieties of dried fruits, candies, lozenges, juice powders, juices, and cosmetics with cranberries.

Product range: almost weekly new outputs

Mouthwash, wash gel for acne and some other personal care products with Vaccinium macrocarpon already exist. The cosmetics industry will come up with even more ideas about the subject of cranberry. Soon it will be just as red as in the food industry. There, the upswing is enormous. Almost every week new products are offered on the world market: jellies, jams, juice blends, compotes, candied or dried berries, fruit slices, sweets, herbal sweets, muesli and fitness bars. However, we better avoid varieties with questionable artificial additives. They are considered to be problematic in intake and utilization. Their molecules are too large to be metabolized by our organism. They often deposit in the fat cells and lead to complaints of organs and blood vessels. That's why we are well advised to spoil our temple body with healthy and nutritious organic products. The processing of organically produced foods prohibits artificial substances such as hydrogenated fats, phosphoric acids, aspartame and monosodium glutamate. These additives are associated with health problems such as heart diseases, osteoporosis, migraine, and hyperactivity (Heaton 2001).

Fresh and frozen cranberries - keepability

We can enjoy the fresh cranberry from the beginning of September to the end of November. You can buy them in 12 oz bags and store them in the refrigerator for three months. In the frozen condition, they should be available all year round. The berries frozen in bulk, go directly from the harvest fields to the freezer. The IQF (Individual Quick Frozen) cranberries are sorted and then individually frozen. The frozen fruits are also offered cut and are versatile, for instance as an ingredient in cake mixtures and sorted according to size. They are of higher quality due to surplus sorting and cleaning.

We can eat the berries fresh with or without cream or serve them in a delicious dish or cake. Or we can treat our inner child by puree the fruit with some cream. Sweetened with stevia or agave juice, we'll get a delicious ice cream in the freezer compartment. Another type of sterilizing is inserting into alcohol. Two tablespoons give each salad, main dish or dessert a special touch.

By the pickling in vinegar, we can free the berry from a bit bitter taste.

Here are other ways to make cranberries durable: we can dry them, juice them, pulp them and freeze them completely or as fruit.

Sirup, concentrate, and powder

In North America, almost every child knows: cranberry juice helps with inflammation of the urinary tract. That's why you find the juice in all food markets and the beverage trade, around the clock. Shops are open every day. In Germany, if the bladder irritates on a Saturday evening, it is useful have frozen small portions of cranberry juice. Then you can quickly conjure up a delicious ice cream:

defrost for 10 minutes, pour into the blender and whisk with a few tablespoons whipped cream and some stevia. If we put the whole large bottle in the refrigerator, the berry juice might get sour. It would be a pity if we had to throw half of it away. It had happened to me before since, when the bladder pain had stopped I'd forgotten and the precious water juice. Today I freeze smaller portions.

The concentrate consists of ground, depectinized cranberries. They are pressed, the juice filtered finely and concentrated under vacuum at low temperature. Essence is added again. Cranberry powder is a pure fruit concentrate with added magnesium citrate or maltose dextrin. It is concentrated under vacuum at low temperatures. The spray drying to 2-5% moisture is performed using tricalcium phosphate as an anti-stick agent. The powder is then examined.

At parties, neither hosts nor guests are disturbed when I make my red wine on the faucet. I just sprinkle powder in the glass, fill water in and marvel at the whitecap and that something so healthy can taste so good. To the cranberry juice from the health food store, I notice no difference. I love sour and bitter. Therefore I mix the powder with water only. If you like it sweeter, you can mix it with apple, mango, cherry or pineapple juice or other fruit juices. Juices, powder or ground cranberries you can buy all year in pharmacies, health food stores or online in international trade. You can thin the 100% juice with three parts of water or sweet juices.

Cranberry powder is offered in small bags, capsules, and cans allowing you to energize almost all dishes, refine creams and keep food fresh longer. Together with the dried berries, other fruits, and ground almonds or nuts, you can make delicious fruit slices. The powder can also be used instead of vinegar for acidifying soups, stews, and salads.

Cranberry juices and juice mixtures

Most of the cranberries are processed into fresh juice, juice mixes or concentrate immediately after harvesting. Today, in every well-stocked beverage and food market, we find products in which the cranberry provides color and freshness. The most famous cocktail is the *Cranberry Classic* from Oceanspray. At the beginning of 2007, US operations will also launch a light product.

The health food store offers delicious organic products: apple juice, apple cherry, bitter lemon and ginger lemonade with cranberry alternatively sweetened of course. Also, I found a cranberry-mix drink with ginkgo. The beverages traders offer dark red organic sodas as a sparkling alternative to the red wine: mineral water, cassis, and cranberry juice - not a bit sweet, like dry vine juice, and quite cheap. So just ask for the health-promoting organic sodas with the trend berry at bars receptions and candlelight dinners. It does not always have to be wine.

Because of the slight tart flavor, cranberry juice is mostly combined with other ingredients. Only the pure mother juice (pharmacy, health food store) is produced without sweet additions and can be mixed with natural fruit juices. In chapters, Cranberry mixtures and Cocktails & Dreams you find cranberry juice mixed with exciting drinks.

Cranberry dry fruits & snacks

Sweetened, dried cranberries contain slightly more than a third of fruit solids thus their positive health properties. The fruits are non-sulphurised and free of dyes. Their sweet-sour taste makes them a fine complement to a variety of recipes. The unique red color excellently accentuates soups, salads, main dishes, cakes, and desserts. Sweetened and dried cranberries are produced by inserting a sucrose sirup into the sliced fruits until a balanced Brix-Grad (sugar content/concentration) is achieved. Then, water is removed from the cranberries until the necessary degree of moisture is reached. They are slightly sprinkled with sunflower oil. Health products contain agave sirup but are about twice as expensive. Whoever wants to have the berries, like myself unsweetened, can dry the fresh oneself.

You can already buy dried cranberries in almost all food markets, health food stores, health food stores and kiosks. At least, however, energy bars and fruit slices, which contain large cranberries besides cherry juice, apples or other fruits. Also in muesli and pastries you will find the red healer. I wish you a lot of fun!

Whoever wants to have the berries, like myself unsweetened, can dry the fresh oneself.

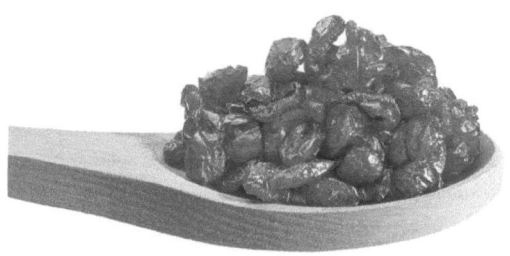

Nutritional analysis of cranberry products (per 100 g)

Nutrient	Frozen a)	Concentrate	Sweetened dried b)	Flavored pieces c)	Powder
Calories	48	198	298 - 367	337 – 342	360
Calories from fat	0	0	11 – 12	5	2
Total fat, g	0,5	0	1,2 – 1,4	0,5	0,2
Saturated fatty acids, g	0	0	0	0	0
Cholesterol, mg	0	0	0	0	0
Sodium, mg	3	14	3 – 4	2 – 3	29
Potassium, mg	73	500	40 – 90	11	734
Carbohydrates, g	10	49	82 – 88	83 – 84	89
Fiber, g	4	<0,5	6 – 9	5 – 6	6
Sugar, g	4	22	64 – 69	67 – 68	37
Protein, g	0,6	<0,5	<0,5	<0,5	<0,5
Vitamin A, IU d)	0	0	70 e)	16,200 f)	0
Vitamin C, mg	18	58	0	1	5
Calcium, mg	10	39	10 – 18	4	184
Iron mg	0,6	1,7	0,5	0	4

a) Whole or in slices
b) Quality: uniform, soft & moist, with glycerine
c) Fruit pieces with peach, bilberry, cherry, strawberry or raspberry flavor
d) Provitamin A
e) Value for sweetened dried cranberries with glycerine. Uniform soft & moist qualities contain 0 I.U.
f) Value for fruit pieces with an orange and peach flavor. Other flavors contain 0 I.U.

Source: American Institute of Baking Technical Bulletin. Volume XXII, December 12, 2000 edition.

Acid fruits conquer the media

Cranberry has been making headlines in 2006. A year later, it conquered Europe by storm. In pharmacies and natural cosmetics, the business flourishes with the red berry. Cranberry juice is already on everyone's lips, because of its positive effect against bacteria.

The TV series Sex in the City has provided for all sorts of talking stuff. And by the way, it has introduced the cranberries to us: cranberry juice and sirup are important ingredients for a Cosmopolitan (see recipe), the favorite cocktail of the main actress. Less public is the special healing powers which are in the cranberry.

This is why the Bonn-based company mk² carried out an extensive media campaign on behalf of the *Cranberry Marketing Committee*. Browsing through the fitness magazines, the vitamin bombs of the food spots are mouthwatering crispy red. More than 200 articles and a lot of TV contributions were devoted to the berries. From the cooking pages of the Gourmet magazine, it glows ruby red.

Health and wellness magazines praise the relative of the cowberry. The trend berry is outpacing its European cousin. The fresh acidity of the cranberry delights the palate more than the more dominant cranberry, the top chef Tim Raue from the Berlin Restaurant 44 in the Berlin Tagesspiegel expresses. When eating and drinking, cranberries belong to a festive menu, best in a composition in red: In the fruit tart and the shallot confit, they are not just a taste highlight.

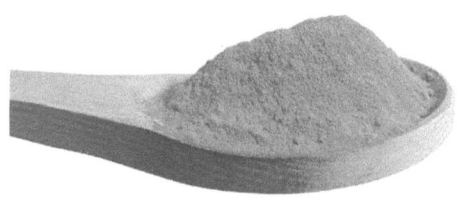

Superpower against bacteria

The editorial department for health in *Frau im Spiegel* does not make the decision for its readers: antibiotics - yes or no? Yet, they recommend "kidney and bladder tea, plenty of water and cranberry juice" as a self-medication. Another tabloid praises the berries as a "super weapon for urinary tract infections and to protect the stomach mucosa and the gums" recommending the fresh fruit or juice. Christine Golli likes to use the fresh berries in her cooking studio, during the winter months: the herb-fruity power berries are healthy and taste delicious as a compote to game dishes.

The drug store recommends the regular consumption of the unsweetened juice to prevent plaque formation and prevent caries. The *Viva* magazine presented an exotic tasting drink: cranberry juice, ginger, honey and kombucha drink on ice: for detoxification.

In the 1920s, researchers discovered drinking cranberry juice makes the urine acidic. It is known the urinary tract-infection bacteria *E. coli* dislike an acidic milieu. Physicians concluded to have found a scientific explanation for the traditional uses of cranberry leading to general medical use of cranberry juice for treating bladder infections.

In the early 1950th the American cranberry was even researched as a medium for speedy detachment of nits from the hair. But extensive studies have focused on the preventive effects of *Vaccinium macrocarpon* against urinary tract infections. In a more recent study, Jiadong Sun and his colleagues from the US University of Rhode Island found out that a cranberry fraction reduced biofilm production by the uropathogenic Escherichia coli CFT073 strain by over 50%. Their results suggest that cranberry oligosaccharides, additionally to its phenolic constituents, may play a role in its preventive effects against urinary tract infections (Jiadong Sun et al 2015).

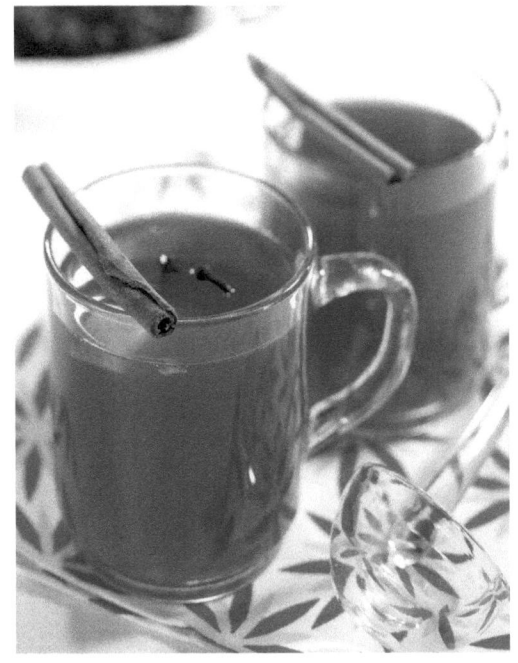

III. FACTS AND FOLKLORE

The cranberry botanized

American Cranberry
(Vaccinium macrocarpon)

Scientific classification

Kingdom:	Plantae
(unranked):	Angiosperms
(unranked):	Eudicots
(unranked):	Asterids
Order:	Ericales
Family:	Ericaceae
Genus:	*Vaccinium*
Subgenus:	**Oxycoccus**

Species
Vaccinium erythrocarpum
Vaccinium macrocarpon
Vaccinium microcarpum
Vaccinium oxycoccos

https://en.wikipedia.org/wiki/Cranberry

Cranberry belongs to the family of heather plants (Ericaceae), subspecies Oxycoccus (common cranberry / Vaccinium oxycoccos). It differs from the other Vaccinium species by means of four-petaled flowers with back-thrown petals. It is diploid, thus having a double chromosome set (2 n = 24). The egg-shaped fruit is cherry-to-olive-sized and is in ripe condition usually of bright red color. The berry has a bright, crunchy solid flesh and a fruity taste. Their natural spread is limited to North America. In the USA, cultivation is mainly restricted to the states of Wisconsin, Massachusetts, New Jersey, Oregon and Washington. In 2016 more than 1.2 million tons of cranberries were harvested. According to a Bulletin of the Agricultural Experimental Station of the University of Massachusetts, there are 175 different cranberry varieties. Most are readings from wild animals and bear the names of the farmers who have selected them including *The Big Four* :

The **Early Black** was named in 1875 in Massachusetts. It is the most frequently cultivated breed. The medium-sized, black-red shining and pear-shaped berry is ripe from the beginning of September. Change the storage results of the variety suitable for many types of soil. The returns are only mediocre. Because of its dark color, it is good for the production of juice and compote to use well.

The **Howes** got its name in 1843 in Massachusetts. It is mature not until October and therefore of little use for northern cultivation areas. Up to 23 mm long it is oval, uniformly large, medium red, shining and maturing well on the bearing. Thanks to its high pectin content, it gelatinizes more and can, therefore, be used well. It is storable and profitable.

The **Mc Farlin** was selected in 1874 in Massachusetts and is the main variety in Washington and the Pacific States. This cranberry is ready to harvest in the middle of October. It is long-rounded, non-uniform, up to 27 mm in size, profitable and deep red with a strong hoop (wax layer). Firm and durable it is of good quality.

The selection of the **Searles** (Jumbo) took place in Wisconsin in 1893. It is the headquarters there and reaches its full maturity in the second half of September. The berry is up to 23 mm in size, is langoval, deep red, also spotted and without gloss. It looks similar to the red mini plum growing in our garden. The Searles is very productive, storable and of good quality. It has the highest vitamin C content (38.2 mg per 100 g) compared to its species and the other cranberry readings.
www. Cranberries.de/70.0.html)

Most of the harvest comes from the US states of Wisconsin, Massachusetts, New Jersey, Oregon and Washington, as well as from the Canadian states of British Columbia and Quebec.

Habitat requirements

Cranberries thrive only on soils with a pH between 4.0 and 5.0. In the USA, mooring with a sandy soil is preferred for cultivation. The plants love a climate with humid-cool summers and mild winters with temperatures down to -18 ° C. In the case of prolonged periods of cold, the leaves may dry out. Then the fields must be flooded. Areas are needed, which allow the water to drain quickly. At the same time, however, they should be able to be overloaded with water in a few hours 7 to 10 cm high in order to avoid frost damage. However, longer flooding tolerates the plants badly. Therefore, the water should be able to drain again quickly.

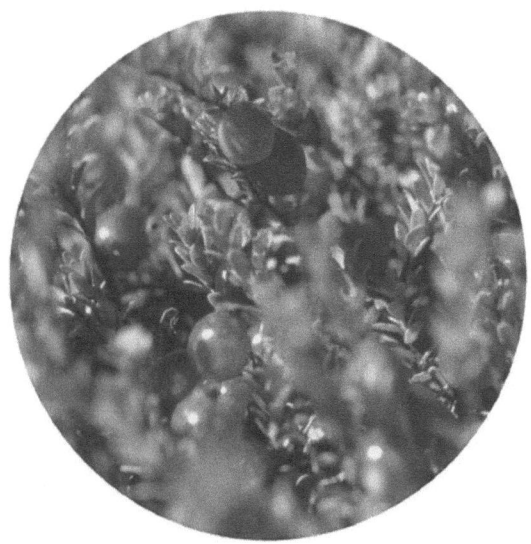

Growth process of the capricious roots

The cranberries growing at low bushes place high demands on soil and climate. They thrive only on very acid high-mountain soils, require a lot of water and a favorable climate in which they can mature from May to October. Ideal conditions for commercial cultivation include, in addition to the already mentioned main cultivation areas, the US states of Connecticut, Michigan, Minnesota, New York and Rhode Island.

At www.cranberries.de/70.0.html botany I found the following statement: Cranberries have adapted with their plant cultivation to the conditions of their location. The plants have the ability to form short secondary roots on their sprouts but do not develop a rootstock. Since I happened to be sitting next to an agricultural scientist in the Gospel choir, I'd contacted her. Dr. Renate Kaiser-Alexnat also found it unusual that the plant should not form a rootstock. She could not find anything in her books and on the Internet. So I called around a bit in the States and landed at the *UMass Cranberry Experiment Station*. Carolyn Demoranvilli told me that there is no rootstock as on an apple tree. The plant has a 5-15 cm deep underground stem but no root hairs. It is a kind of fibrous mat (fiber root). The wooden structure resembles that of a vine stock.

The shoots grow almost endlessly and form roots in contact with the soil. The cranberry grows up to two meters in length, on the ground. Its runners make cranberries the record holder among the relatives of their species. The side roots on the shoots are short and unbranched. As mentioned, they do not form root-hairs, as all the plants of the heather family comprising about 50 species.

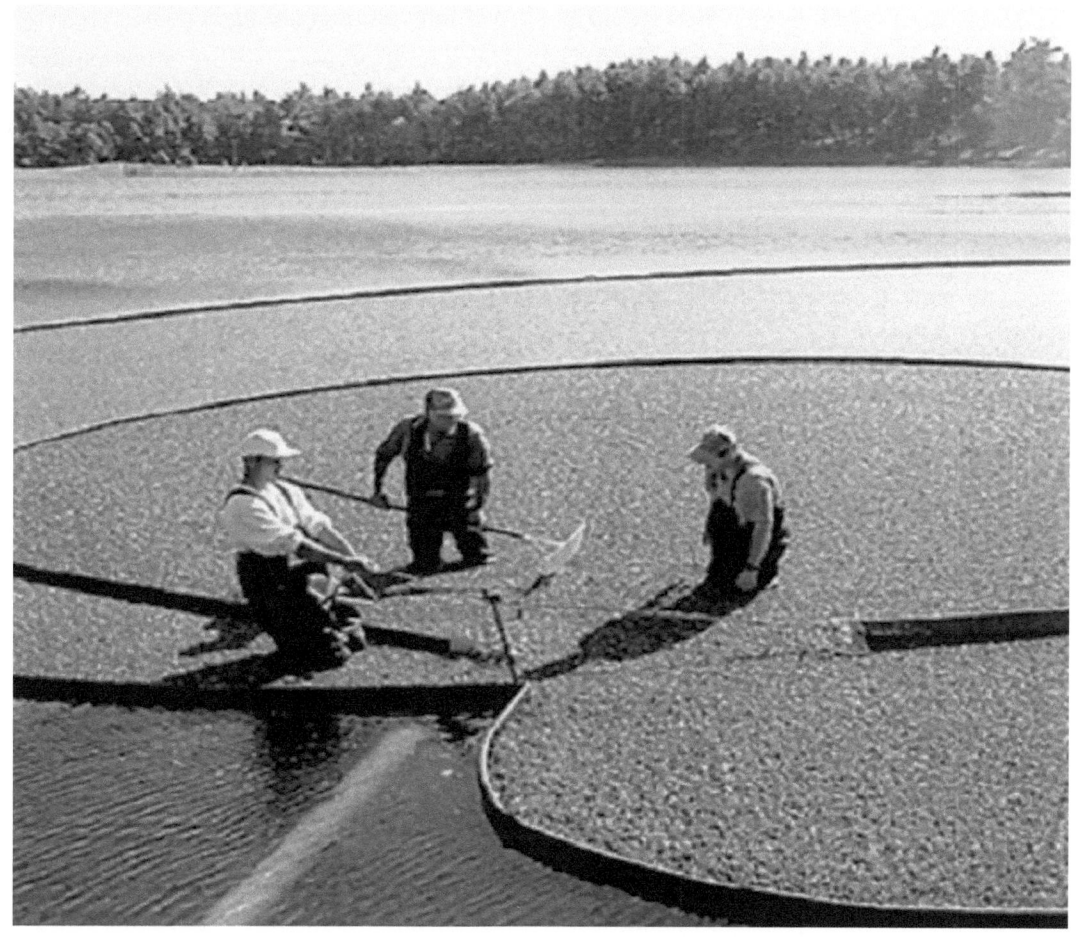

They rather depend on the symbiotic relationship with mycorrhizal fungi, enabling them to thrive on extremely acid soils.

In May the plants awaken from their winter sleep. First, new leaves develop on the long vines which are growing above the ground. From mid-June, the magnificent pink flowers bloom. After three to six weeks, they are faded. Then there are tiny green knots growing to cranberries in the course of the summer. It takes 2½ to 3½ months until the berries have fully developed. In September and October, they reach their full maturity. The red color is formed when the temperature is very low. In November the leaves on the harvested shrubs become red too. Then the fruits of the harvest of the following year begin to form. To protect this crop over the winter most cranberry fields are also flooded in the winter. This way, the fruit mixtures, which are then submerged, do not suffer frost damage. The frozen surfaces are strewn with sand during the winter, as a cranberry farmer in the middle of the last century found out by chance:

Cranberries sprinkled with sand become bigger and juicier.

The Harvest of cranberry: a berry sports festival

Though I've visited five typical cranberry states, mostly at harvest time from near I've never witnessed the picking of the red splendor. However, I hope to be able to collect my own experience on one of the colorful events one of the next falls.

The farmers today apply two different methods of harvesting:

Dry harvest: when berries are jumping

The *Paradise Meadow* cranberry is harvested in this labor-intensive way since 1935, near Cape Cod, Massachusetts. In the dry harvest, the workers have to wait until the dew has dried on the branches starting harvesting, not before 10 o'clock in the morning. 35 to 40 harvesters pick up about 36,000 kilos of the precious berries within one day with picking machines similar to lawnmowers. They are hand-picked or collected with comb-like conveyor belts and packaged in linen bags or barrels. They then come to the collection stations and are tested for color and strength.

The last test is about the jumping power of the cranberries. They have to jump seven times over ten centimeters high wooden barriers. Damaged, soft berries do not manage the test jumping and are sorted out.

As early as the end of the 19th century, the first machine was developed, which works according to this principle of quality control. The whole cranberries go on sale as fresh fruits or are for export. After the dry harvest, the cultivation areas are flooded for a week in order to grow torn shoots again and collect fallen berries and torn plant parts on the shore.

Wet harvest: swimming is cool

The largest portion of US production (95%) is harvested wet which is far less expensive. The farmer floods the cranberry fields up to 45 cm high. Artificially generated water vortex dissolve the berries from the shrubs. Each one contains four air chambers. Therefore, the cranberries swim on the water surface and only have to be picked up. This way, only six workers harvest about 136,000 kilos in one day destined for further processing into juice, jelly or powder. The peeled off berries are collected with the machine or in a corner of the watering place.

With older systems, scoops are used to comb out the fruit. Additionally, today multifunctional harvesting machines work in dry or flooded systems. Wet harvesting farmers are often chipping the berries. The wind blows them to the shore. They are filled with conveyor belts into transport containers. Wet harvested cranberries are mainly put to industrial use.

History and mystery

The health-promoting properties of cranberry have long been known in the USA and are part of folk traditions. Hundreds of years before the colonists came, the Native Americans already appreciated them as medicines and food. They processed the berries with deer meat to a feast. When Indian tribes gathered at festivals cranberries were served as a gesture of peace and friendship. These fruits growing in vines in the sandy Moorland of southeastern Massachusetts are said to have been handed over to the first Thanksgiving of the pilgrims with the chief Massasoit. In 1621 the immigrants were still at peace with the natives of the Wampanoags tribe. David E. Stannard has described it in his book *American Holocaust: The Conquest of the*

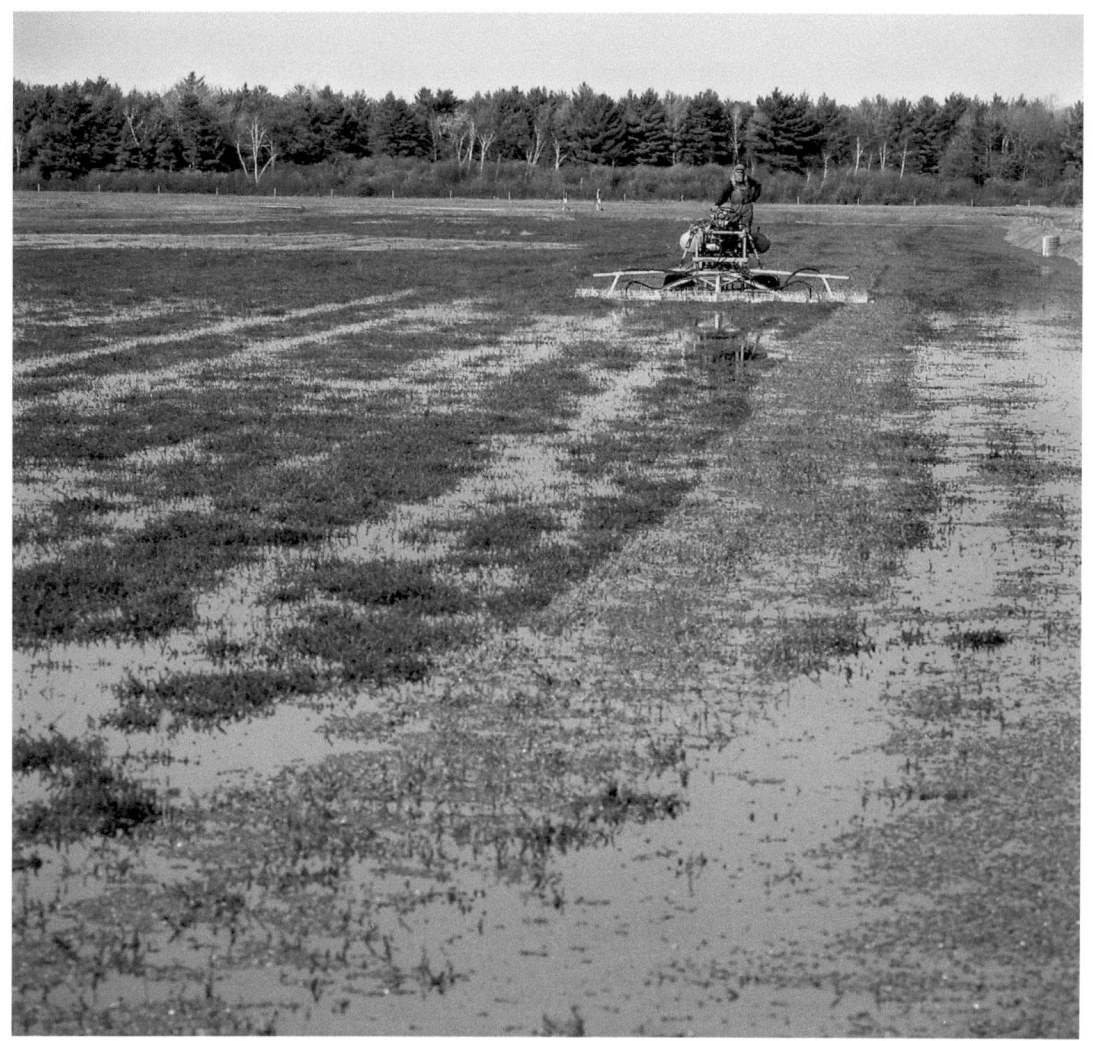

New World. But don't worry, I'm not going to dig up the gloomy chapter of the first decades of the British colonial foundations in North America. Although Germans my generation seem to be predestined for looking back on and reviewing horror history. In my experience report *Family Code*, I showed people depend on different traditions (2017).

The Indians used the cranberry juice with a natural disinfecting effect as a preservative. With the "ibimi" or "bitter berry" as the Pequots and the Leni-Lenape tribes named the cranberry they dyed their woolen blankets and fabrics. They also used the sour fruits to heal wounds: with the help of cranberry packs, they pulled poison from their arrows. And because they are so long lasting because of their natural wax layer, American sailors took them in large quantities into wooden barrels on their sea voyages. In the case of whale exploration or the exploration of China, the vitamin C-containing fruit helped to prevent the scarring disease scurvy. Already during the 17th century, the following healing effects of the cranberry were documented: It helps with blood disorders, stomach problems, liver problems, vomiting, appetite deficit, scurvy, and cancer.

www.herbalgram.org

Today the berries are known for their essential phytochemicals and are therefore recommended for strengthening the defenses. Regular consumption of cranberries reduces the risk of urinary tract diseases, reduces the risk of tooth decay and caries and strengthens the immune system.

Usage: a good fit with cranberries

With their intense fruit flavor, the bright red nutrient bombs provide variety in the daily diet: as a snack, the dry fruits quickly provide energy curbing frequent sugar cravings. As a cooking ingredient, they add a special touch to all kinds of dishes. Also with baking, cranberries offer a wide range of uses. Their slightly herbal fruit aroma harmonizes with many dishes with light or dark meat and fish. In vegetable dishes, fruit salads or sweets the berries provide variety. With their appealing, invigorating and activating effect, they set new accents. Fresh or freshly pressed, they energize every dish and drink.

Tip: Dried fruits soaked for 2 to 3 hours in cranberry or other fruit juice, can be used like fresh fruits. Bananas or melons I would not eat together with the sour fruit. Otherwise, almost all food fit it. For preparing your cereal, soak the dried berries in a bowl with the cereals, the seeds, germs, nuts or apple pieces overnight in almond, oat, or rice milk. And as I said, if sugar is problematic, you can dry or freeze the fresh berries available in autumn.

A delicious snack: cranberry powder in sheep yogurt. Experimenting with the berry, I found out that with it nearly all main dishes and desserts can be refined. Particularly popular are the juicy muffins and pastries with cranberries.

Monika Helmke Hausen writes about the little cousin in her book *Die Botschaft der Früchte*: "...oranges, and almonds strengthen and support the principle of the cowberry in a perfect way." This refers to the creative idea and the determination of the fruit: To help people in their search for themselves, to promote the education of the homeland and to help others to forgive themselves and others.

If bladder problems are a topic in our lives, it means that the soul does not feel well.

For that, the berry stimulates the center of the soul and also the thyroid gland, "so that the self-consciousness comes gently, but surely expresses" (p. 265).

Awaken cranberries the *joie de vivre* of the cow?

Whose mouth does not water while looking at the red ripe berries in the culinary part of relevant magazines? They seem to awaken a sense of life and courage. The Funk & Wagnalls New Encyclopedia also mentions the lingonberry or cowberry (Vaccinium vitis-idaea) as a wild-growing relative of the cranberry in the subarctic regions of Canada and in the alpine regions of North America or Northern Europe, also called the mountain cranberry. How did the name cowberry come about? Perhaps a sick ruminant got well by chewing the berries. Or had a farmer exchanged his cow for a piece of land with cranberry plants? Or had a sad cow enjoyed life again with the berry?

Another variety of berries is the highbush cranberry (*Viburnum opulus*) sometimes used as a substitute for the cranberry. Concentrated white blossoms are followed by red fruits. The Flora list of Baden-Wuerttemberg still points to the northern bilberry as a heather plant and assigns it to the type Vaccinium uliginosum.

The taste of chocolate has long been the first priority of our taste buds. Berries follow. But about the encouraging effect of cranberry, we only know for several years. Today we do not even have to wait for the fall since we can buy enough cranberry products all year round. These can always be energized with some fresh organic lemon juice.

In comparison with the cowberry

Botanists of yesterday and today may argue about the cultivation areas of the Vaccinium macrocarpon. One thing is for sure: The olive-sized ruby berry is rooted in the northern part of the USA and in Canada. Cranberries grow on 10 to 20 cm high shrubs with long soil vines. They stand out by their exquisite pink-white flowers. The cranberries ripen on upright dwarf shrubs and have bell-shaped downwards open flowers. The leaves are broadly obtuse ovate shining at the top. The cranberry prefers sandy, humus moderately acidic soil. Their minor pulp contains a large number of small seeds.

Does the Eurasian cousin of the cranberry have the same properties to keeping the urinary tract and the bladder healthy? Similar characteristics I would suspect. But they were primarily found in cranberry. The contents of both berries also vary. The cranberry contains more iron and vitamin C than the lingonberry. Cranberry juice is used for a long time in the USA against bladder infections and urinary tract infections due to antiviral, bactericidal and fungicidal active ingredients. The fresh acidity of the cranberry delights the palate more than the more dominant cowberry. Whether the amount or composition of arbutin, quinic acid, hippuric acid, and tannin is responsible for the more severe flavor may remain unaffected. Even if the larger trend berry is preferred, you may test the cowberry as well. On the Frisian island of Terschelling, the best cowberry of the world should grow. Why not re-explore the old acid fruit?

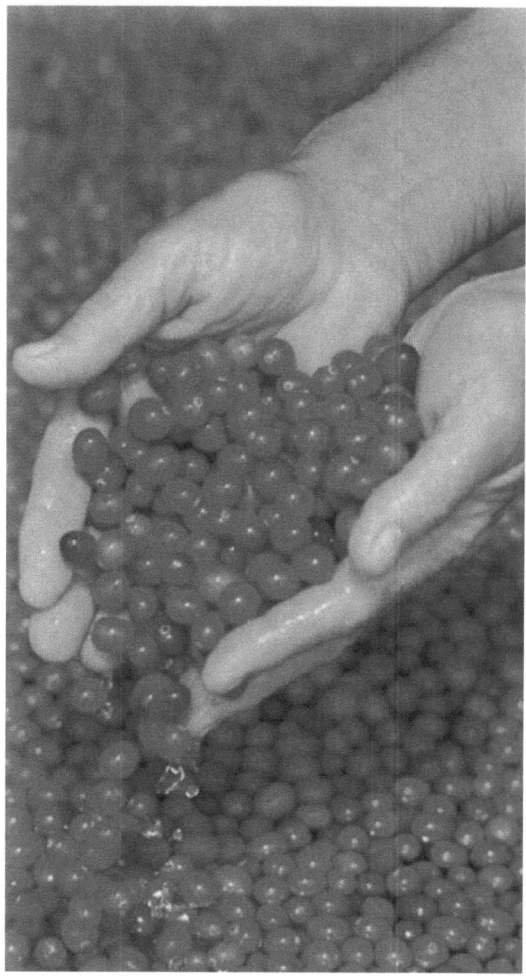

IV. HEALTH ENHANCING CONTENTS

What's in the redskin?

With this question, I got to work on the list of vital substances. Compare to the analysis of Spirulina platensis the Vaccinium macrocarpon looks poorly. I've dedicated a dissertation and seven books to the blue-green microorganism because it's a great source of vital substances.

But when I studied the cranberry I was impressed with the results confirming its remarkable healing power. "A review of cranberry research targeting cancer revealed positive effects of cranberries or cranberry derived constituents against 17 different cancers utilizing a variety of in vitro techniques, whereas in vivo studies supported the inhibitory action of cranberries toward cancers of the esophagus, stomach, colon, bladder, prostate, glioblastoma, and lymphoma." (Weh et al. 2016)

The cranberry is also promising in the no. 1 Killer heart and circulatory diseases and the associated arteriosclerosis.

It is less the vitamins and minerals, but above all the secondary plant substances that make the acid fruit so valuable:

Secondary metabolites: Can we reverse the clock?

Phytochemicals are natural substances controlling growth. Plants produce these bioactive substances as protection against pests. As colorants and fragrances, they attract pollen-spreading insects and seed-spreading fruit-eaters. But man too can benefit from them. In the past, we combine the protective groups, which are mainly in the colors, with a healthy diet or health-promoting effect. For a long time, we know that vegetables, fruits, nuts, sprouted seeds, and legumes are good for us. But so far the experts have assumed that only vitamins, minerals, and fiber are responsible for it. Meanwhile, researchers have discovered a cornucopia of the most powerful antioxidants.

If we eat many different colored natural foods, our organism utilizes these disease-preventing phytochemicals optimally.

They also play an increasingly important role as preparations or functional foods. Juices and snacks are now no longer only beefed up with proteins, minerals, vitamins, and beneficial bacteria, but also with phytochemicals. The prospect of staying healthy and vital to the old age, without having to carefully select the fresh ingredients and to have to deal with them, let many consumers resort to designer food. I doubt the investment of these expensive foods pays off. They do not substitute a balanced diet. With the "ibimi" or "bitter berry" as the P

As long as the secondary metabolites and antioxidants occur naturally in fruits, vegetables, and herbs their positive effects are undisputed. But in the artificially enriched food with phytochemicals, the interplay and interactions of the substances have not yet been explored. To be on the safe side, we better remain with the products given to us by creation.

We do not need to worry about whether the amount and mix are right or violate our temple. Only substances bound to the plant are attributed to a cancer risk reducing or cancer preventive function. Only these are known to protect the body from fungi, bacteria, and viruses. And only from flavonoids, polyphenols, and carotenoids bound to the plant, we know that they are antioxidants and stimulate the immune system.

How do the phytochemicals work?

Secondary plant substances catch free radicals associated with many diseases rendering them harmless and reducing oxidative stress. It is known that the oxidative stress caused by reactive oxygen-containing intermediates damages the cells: oxygen binds in the body with hydrogen atoms to water. A large portion of this water is excreted through the urinary tract. This combustion process increases the energy of the body. Since free radicals have an unpaired electron, they are highly unstable. In the pursuit of the noble gas configuration, they try to acquire the missing electron. They attack and alter neighboring molecules: fats, proteins or DNA.

Secondary plant compounds not only protect our cells from oxidation and thus from premature aging. They also enhance the efficiency of all other antioxidants,

such as vitamins A, C, and E. These, in turn, neutralize the cell-damaging effect of free radicals in the body. They inhibit the development of cancer and thrombosis, strengthen the immune system and positively influence the blood glucose and cholesterol levels. Thus the phytochemical diseases can prevent and cure diseases.

Oligomeric procyanidins (OPC) or proanthocyanidins (PAC)

OPC or PAC are a biochemical group of substances occurring in plants belonging to the group of flavanols. Proanthocyanidins: authors = flower, cyanidin (magenta). "Anthocyanins are the red or blue dyestuffs of the higher plants which are always dissolved in the cell juice. They are nitrogen-free and rich in oxygen "(Küster 1920, p. 196).

Since 1983 OPC has been investigated with regard to its antioxidative functions and its use in preventing disease. The OPC of maritime coniferous trees and grape cores was considered especially effective demonstrating a very strong antioxidative (protective) effect against free radicals.

Cranberries contain a variety of secondary metabolites. They slow down the cell oxidation and are effective in the blood vessels: dilut the blood, lower the LDL cholesterol and the blood pressure, dilate the vessels and have an anti-inflammatory effect. So cranberry may prevent fatty deposits (plaques) in the blood vessels.

US researchers found out that cranberries work against arterial calcification and inhibit cancer.

How many antioxidants do we consume?

When we drink red wine, we take in around 30 mg per 100 ml. Particularly in the summer months, the fruitarian's intake can often rise to several hundred milligrams daily by the more frequent consumption of berry fruits. It is estimated that 10% of the population does not eat any red, violet or blue plants at all. The U.S. Department of Agriculture examined the total content of PAC and OPC of various fruits. The researchers found that cranberries with 418.8 mg/100g had the highest concentration of these also called condensed tannins followed by wildly growing blueberries with 331.9, plums 215.9, blueberries from agricultural cultivation with 179.8 and strawberries with 145.0.

Researchers from Cornell University, Ithaca, New York, found the highest proportion of health-promoting phenols in fruits in cranberry. This confirms its cancer prevention effect (San et al. 2002).

Polyphenol comparison of beverages

(Total polyphenol content in 237 ml - 8 oz.)

Cranberry juice 587 mg
Red wine 400 mg
Grape juice 356 mg
Cranberry juice cocktail 137 mg
Apple juice 61 mg
Orange juice 53 mg

Polyphenol comparison of foods
(Food per serving)

Red grape (140 g) 518 mg
Cranberry (55 g) 373 mg
Whole milk chocolate (30 g) 296 mg
Green Grape (140 g) 271 mg
Apple (140 g) 260 mg
Banana (140) 193 mg
Blueberry (55 g) 186 mg
Strawberry (140 g) 144 mg
Broccoli (85 g) 89 mg
Orange (140 g) 58 mg

The information in the two tables is from the brochure "Technical Information for the Food Industry" (*CMC Cranberry Marketing Committee*). The CMC represents the cranberry industry in the USA, ensuring a balance between supply and demand and promoting the use and consumption of fruits in the USA, Japan, Germany, and Mexico.

PAC or OPC is found primarily in the kernels and outer layers of many fruits, peanuts, and some vegetable and herbal varieties. Berries contain most of this substance group.

The health effects of red wine confirmed in many studies are presumably due to the high content of OPC. Like cranberry, red wine contains a number of other essential plant substances, so the effects add up.

Health effects of PAC/OPC

- protects against oxidative stress
- strengthens cardiovascular functions
- protects against high blood pressure
- strengthens the digestive system
- supports eye functions
- strengthens the immune system
- prevents edema formation
- protects the fragile capillaries and reduces their permeability
- protects against excessive collision of blood platelets (lowering of the thrombosis risk)
- inhibits the skin aging process by activating or forming collagen
- facilitates the light adjustment of the eye from gleaming to sepulchral darkness
- supports the retina and is recommended in the case of nearsightedness
- strengthens the immune system: protects cell changes and inflammation
- promotes the functions of vitamin C and helps in the recycling of vitamin E
- is designed as an antioxidant against hydroxyl radicals as well as against lipid peroxidation and reduces thereby the deposition of oxidized LDL cholesterol in the blood vessel walls
- protects the liver cells from damage by painkillers
- protects the DNA

PAC/OPC as food additives

This group of substances is very well tolerated and permitted as food additives (E163, dyes without quantitative limits). OPC is relatively poorly bio-available when taken orally. The intake from the gastrointestinal tract is approximately 5 percent. However, this amount is sufficient to achieve the desired health effects. After exposure, the plasma levels increase rapidly and decrease within two hours. Water soluble OPC is much more bio-available. It is transported across the blood to all organs and tissues and passes the blood-brain barrier.

Lutein and zeaxanthin prevent macular degeneration

100 ml of cranberry juice contains 68 mcg of these carotenoids. These are antioxidants that are ten times more effective than vitamin E.

Their yellow pigments filter harmful UV rays and blue light from sunlight. This reduces the risk of macular degeneration and cataract. The yellow-orange xanthophyll lutein is next to the beta carotene the most widely used carotenoid. Researchers from around the world confirm the correlation between AMD and low carotenoid concentrations. The visual acuity increased in a study, especially in blue-eyed persons.

(Dagnelie, 2000). In addition, Bone and colleagues were able to show in the living and the deceased: AMD patients show a significantly lower lutein and zeaxanthin concentration in the macula (2000, 2001). See the chapter DISEASES PREVENTION AND HEALING FROM A - Z under macular degeneration.

Overall, secondary plant substances prevent and cure diseases by strengthening the immune system by intensifying the effects of antioxidants. To protect us from health problems, we better eat a lot of fruit, especially berries. In the poor fruit season, we can drink cranberry juice and other berry juices. If you eat muesli in the morning, you can spread dried berries or cranberry powder over it. You find numerous other possibilities to use cranberries and berry juice in the culinary section.

Vitamin C - ascorbic acid – E 300

This water-soluble antioxidant also prevents harmful reactions in blood and cell fluids. It is used in food production and found as E 300 in ingredients lists. Most experts report vitamin C requirements for women with 75 mg, for men with 90 mg. According to the literature, the cranberry has a vitamin C content of 7.5 to 13 mg per 100 g. However, there are also data on fresh berries which are around 29 mg. The Searles (Jumbo) should even contain 38 mg.

Average analysis of cranberry juice

Water	g	87.13
Energy	kcal	46
Energy	kJ	194
Protein	g	0.39
Total lipids (fat)	g	0.13
Minerals (ash)	g	0.15
Carbohydrates	g	12.20
Dietary fiber	g	0.1
Total sugar	g	12.10

Minerals

Calcium, Ca	mg	8
Iron, Fe	mg	0.25
Magnesium, Mg	mg	6
Phosphorus, P	mg	13
Potassium, K	mg	77
Sodium, Na	mg	2
Zinc, Zn	mg	0.10
Copper, Cu	mg	0.055
Selenium, Se	mcg	0.1

Vitamins

Vitamin C, ascorbic acid	mg	9.3
Vitamin B1 (thiamine)	mg	0.009
Vitamin B2 (riboflavin)	mg	0.018
Vitamin B3 (niacin)	mg	0.052
Folate DFE (Dietary Folate Equivalent)	mcg	1
Vitamin A,	IU	45
Provitamin A (retinol)	mcg	2

Vitamin E (alpha-tocopherol) mg		1.20
Vitamin K (phylloquinone)	mcg	5.1

Lipids

Fatty acids, saturated	g	0.010
Fatty acids, monounsaturated	g	0.023
Fatty acids, polyunsaturated	g	0.070
Beta-carotene	mcg	27
Lutein + Zeaxanthin	mcg	68

USDA National Nutrient Database for Standard Reference, Release 18 (2005)

IV. DISEASE PREVENTION AND CURE FROM A - Z

Health disorders are usually due to the poisoning of the body. Pollutants in the food, addiction behavior, drugs, and stress constantly stresses our physical and mental-spiritual milieu. Quite apart from the influence of ionizing radiation, radio waves, electromagnetic and high frequent radiation or electric smog. The allergy and cancer rates, risen drastically in recent years, indicate that the desecration of our temple with toxic substances has become intolerable. Our immune system is constantly challenged to eliminate harmful substances, fight off microbes and destroy cancer cells. The red berry proven to strengthen the immune system and known for a long time in the US as a cure for urinary tract infections has now also been shown effective in numerous other diseases.

Recent scientific studies demonstrate the health-promoting properties of cranberry. Its contents help to maintain a healthy body. Those who regularly enjoy the American cranberry and their products have significantly fewer problems with the urinary and the gastrointestinal tract. Researchers have already taken a closer look at the acidic fruit. In doing so, they discovered rosy gums with a constantly consumed diet of cranberries. Also, a significant reduction of plaque bacteria was observed reducing the risk of caries and periodontal disease. In addition,

the antioxidants of the cranberry delay the ravages of the time and inhibit the growth of cancer cells.

I was especially astonished by the study of some veterinarians, according to which the trend berry could even turn off the No.1 killer: heart and circulatory diseases.

Pigs with calcified arteries had flexible blood vessels after a 6 months daily consumption of cranberry powder

as explained below.

So if you want to spoil your body and keep it healthy, you can cherish it with cranberries. The following is an overview of health problems, which the miracle fruit can influence favorably. This list is, of course, not complete. In recent years, globally the cranberry was studied extensively. To show them all would be beyond the scope of this book.

Arteriosclerosis: stretching for the veins

Cardiac and circulatory diseases cause most people to die. In April 2005, Kris Kruse-Elliott and her colleagues in San Diego reported on the results of their study: Cranberries can make arteriosclerosis vessels elastic again. The researchers at the University of Wisconsin-Madison School of Veterinary Medicine investigated the effect of regular consumption of cranberry juice powder over 6 months and found the following: The vascular function of genetically modified pigs improved so clearly that the condition of their vessels nearly normalized.

The genetic make-up of the pigs examined by the researchers altered in such a way that they spontaneously develop high blood fat values at the age of about eight months. As a result, the typical plaques form in the vessels of the animals, which reduce the vessel diameter and, at the same time, significantly reduce the elasticity of the vessel walls. These changes are very similar to those in patients with arteriosclerosis. Common consequences include severe bleeding disorders of the legs, coronary heart disease, heart attacks and stroke.

The vessels of the animals were considerably more flexible and elastic than those of their conspecifics who had not been fed with cranberry powder indicating cranberries can make the blood vessels of test animals with high cholesterol levels and arteriosclerosis supple.

It is not yet certain which content is responsible for the effect: antioxidants, flavonoids, polyphenols or other substances. The researchers want to clarify it next. Until a similar effect is observed in humans, they recommend increasing the secondary metabolites in the diet such as cranberries and other fruits and vegetable varieties. This improves the vessel function of people with high cholesterol and arteriosclerosis. Thus they can prevent the consequences of inflexible arteries: heart attack and stroke
(ddp/science.de - Ilka Lehnen-Beyel).

Prof. Dr. Heinz Schilcher recommends buckwheat for the prevention and treatment of arteriosclerosis. Wash and soak the grains in the evening. In the morning, they are ready for the muesli.

You could also germinate part of the grains further. Purchased buckwheat flour is no longer alkaline in contrast to the grains. Therefore, we better grind small portions in the coffee or percussion mill ourselves. Chlorophyll-rich food (grass juices, Spirulina), apples and omega-3 fatty acids from fish oil also improve the flow characteristics of the blood and thus counteract the cholesterol deposition or the calcification of the arteries.

Bear leek, speedwell, mistletoe, and field horsetail are Maria Treben's means of preventing arteriosclerosis.

Bladder infections: Cranberries dispel E. coli bacteria

Typical symptoms of bladder infections are frequent urination, low urine volume, and unpleasant burning sensation. The inflammation of the bladder is usually caused by bacteria. These have an easy job with it when the natural defenses of urethra and bladder are weakened. In some persons, cold feet or sitting on the cool ground, and it has already happened. Female members are most affected. Half of all women suffer from a bladder infection once in their life, almost every fifth woman once a year. It's especially up to the female anatomy. The urethra of the woman is much shorter than that of the man. This allows bacteria to reach the bladder more easily. Under certain circumstances, they even get into the kidneys and can cause renal cell inflammation.

Due to its condensed tannins, the cranberry can uniquely prevent urinary tract infections (UTIs) destroying the attachment mechanism of certain E. coli bacteria. Thus they can no longer adhere to the bladder wall. As a result, even before the bacteria can multiply and trigger an inflammation they are flushed out of the body again.

Only recently, Italian researchers confirmed the preventive effect of a cranberry extract (Anthocran®) in recurring urinary tract infections (UTIs) testing 36 juvenile subjects between 12 and 18 years. Of the group who received 120 mg of cranberry extract standardized for 36 mg of proanthocyanidins for 60 days, 63.1 had no symptoms, while in the placebo group only 23.5 were symptom-free; a convincing proof of the efficacy of Anthocran® (Ledda et al., 2017).

An acquaintance went to her doctor because she had blood in the urine. He gave her an antibiotic. On the next examination, her condition was unchanged. Then the doctor recommended drinking cranberry juice. She ate a whole glass full of cranberries and drank the juice in which they were preserved. Next day the urine was clear. Teas from goldenrod, overmanning, buckhorn and thyme also help to heal the bladder. See also under urinary tract infections and cystitis.

Cancer: Special nutrients delay cancer growth

It will not surprise you when I say: fast food can be fatal! Hot Dogs & Co. increase the risk of pancreatic cancer. Ute Nothlings and her colleague L.N. Colonel conducted a large-scale multiethnic study at the Universities of Hawaii-Los Angeles. This revealed:

Excessive consumption of hot dogs, sausages, and other industrially processed meat products can lead to an increased risk of pancreatic cancer (2006).

In addition to heart diseases, cancer is the second most common cause of death in many countries. The prognosis for patients with carcinomas of the lung, colon, breast or prostate is still gloomy. Conventional therapy is unsatisfactory. On the other hand, it is worthwhile to use therapeutically proven natural cancer-inhibitors also in the sense of the cost savings in the disease sector. Next, to the most researched *Spirulina platensis* in this field cranberries have many of these natural inhibitors that are not even all identified. Already in 2002, B.T. Murphy, C.C. Neto et al. found an anti-tumor activity of a polyphenolic component of Vaccinium macrocarpone.

In 2003, scientists at the University of Massachusetts-Dartmouth used bioactivity-driven fractions of cranberry to determine the identity of certain esters. Hitherto, these triphenoid esters, which have played a role in cancer prevention, have not yet been found in the Vaccinium fruit.

In October 2005, researchers led by Catherine C. Neto discovered a completely new way to prevent metastases, that is, the spread of cancer cells to other parts of the body. Their latest in vitro laboratory tests show: Cranberry proanthocyanidins (PAC) inhibit the growth of lung, intestinal tumors, and leukemia cells. A corresponding study was published in the Journal of Science of Food and Agriculture. Dr. Catherine C. Neto recalls the cancer-resistant abilities of the cranberry PAC to their unique A-shaped structure. Most other fruit types have B-shaped structures.

Resveratrol is another anticancer drug. The natural polyphenolic antioxidant comes mainly in grapes, berries and red wine.

Resveratrol protects indistinctly against various types of cancer. Therefore, M.H. Aziz and colleagues from the University of Wisconsin suggested in July 2003 to tests with chemopreventive natural drugs on humans and animals.

Pressed cranberries (cranberry press cakes) had reduced the growth of cancer in mice in a previous study. There was a decline in metastases and tumors. Therefore, Peter J. Ferguson and his colleagues conducted another test with mice. They carried human breast cancer cells. In total, the hot water extract of the pressed cranberries was tested on eight types of cancer: two prostate and two breast cancers as well as skin, colon, lung, and brain cancer. The result was particularly successful in male prostate tumors dependent on male sex hormones.

At the end of 2005, Sun and Hai Liu conducted a study at Cornell University's US Department of Food Science, Ithaca, New York. They found that cranberry phytochemicals have the ability to inhibit human breast cancer growth. In May 2006, Parry and colleagues investigated the antioxidant and anticancer properties of various fruit juice powders. The seed extract of cranberry had the highest content of alpha-linolenic acid and the lowest fat content. It clearly reduced the proliferation of cancer cells in the colon. Similar effects were observed in the extract of the blackberry and the Chardonnay grape. It is possible that several of the secondary plant compounds abundantly contained in the berries help prevent the spread of cancer cells. Thus, cranberries can positively influence the course of different cancer diseases.

Candida: Cranberry helps to prevent fungi

Urinary tract infections mainly affect women. To avoid antibiotic resistance, after the first inflammation preventive measures are recommended. Cranberry juice or powder have proven to be successful.

Usually, antibiotics are prescribed by the doctor, and the patient is advised to drink as much as possible. If you follow this advice, do not forget: strong chemical substances damage the gut flora. As a rule, doctors fail to prescribe intestinal reconstruction at the same time. So we better provide ourselves with probiotic organisms for the reconstruction of the intestinal flora. In many cases, the infection may be cured with antibiotics in a few days. However, recurring urinary tract infections frequently occur. There is also the risk of kidney involvement. Repeated antibiotic therapies damage the intestinal and vaginal flora. Resistance and chronic mycosis develop. We can prevent these yeast overgrowths if, for example, we drink cranberry juice and/or medicines before and after each sexual intercourse. Howell and Foxman were able to prove this in 2002. They cultivated 39 isolated uropathic Escherichia coli bacteria for 20 minutes in cranberry-proanthocyanidins extract and in the urine of healthy women. This was obtained over twelve hours before and after consumption of 240 ml of cranberry juice. The US researchers from the Rutgers University in Chatsworth, NJ, then examined the bacteria for their ability to attach to isolated uroepithelial cells. The urine after the consumption of cranberry juice prevented the adherence of 80 percent of all bacteria and 79% of all antibiotic-resistant bacteria. On the other hand, the germs drawn in the non-enriched urine could adhere unhindered to the cells. The effect began two hours after drinking the juice and lasted for ten hours. This means that the proanthocyanins in the cranberry prevent the docking of even antibiotic-resistant germs. There is no resistance to cranberry. Therefore, we can save costs through the prevention of the antibiotic-induced Candida albicans fungus.

In addition to cranberry, there are a number of tested natural antifungals: Lapacho tea, grapefruit seed extract, Multiplasan mineral complex 33, colloidal silver, colloidal gold. Fungi feel most comfortable in an acid environment. This is why vegetable foodstuff is so important as its alkalines buffer the acids. Alfalfa, algae, cucumbers, chestnut, dandelion, olives, papaya, Spirulina, and zucchini are notably alkaline. See also chapter The anti-candida diet has many benefits.

Caries: The cranberry can scare away germs

How does caries develop? From sugars, bacteria produce energy with the help of enzymes. In this glycolytic process, aggressive acids are formed as waste products. These remove the minerals from the tooth enamel and dissolve it. Streptococci mutans and the lactobacilli, which are desirable in the small intestine, are among the main causes of caries (www.zahnwissen.de).

If you drink a glass of cranberry juice without sugar after breakfast and dinner you will increase the chances of finishing off the teeth attacking bacteria. In Jerusalem, Weiss and colleagues conducted a study with 59 people. 29 used a cranberry mouthwash daily for 6 weeks. In their saliva, the number of streptococci and other bacteria was significantly lower than in the control group of 30 persons who received a placebo mouthwash. The reduction of plaque bacteria reduces the risk of caries and periodontal disease. By the way, the proven slimming green tea also has a damaging effect on the caries bacterium Streptococcus mutans. That is why I now mix cranberry juice with green tea for even more tooth decay protection.

You can also try the oil-pulling presented by the Russian researcher Dr. Fedor Karach. Every time I do this, my teeth look whiter than before and the mouth feels sheer clean. Whether the periodic oil pulling is something for you and helps to prevent tooth decay, you can test yourself: You take a tablespoon of cold pressed sunflower oil in the morning before breakfast, move it about 15 minutes in the mouth and then spit it into the toilet. The oil is said to draw toxins from the body. In the mouth, it turns into a white, highly toxic liquid, which must not be swallowed.

Cataract: The OPC of the power berry protects the lens

Poison and slag deposits cause a lot of damage, even in the eye lens. If you, as I did in my youth, torment your immune system with a lot of stress, vaccines, anesthetics, x-rays, drugs and paste foods, a cataract can quickly become a reality. My "old age" cataract became apparent after a series of operations and serious diseases at the age of 10 years.

The "valuable cow's milk" can also be the culprit. The calcium, partly destroyed by heating, deposits the body as lime. This can lead to arterial calcification, rheumatism, arthritis, osteoporosis and kidney stones. I am not writing this for the first time. I often talk about this with relatives and friends or give them my books. However, they continue to drink milk and continue to suffer from rheumatoid arthritis, osteoporosis, mucous congestion and more. Only one of my friends had taken action. She already had distinct deformations on her finger joints. After changing her diet she got rid of the deformations.

The clouding of the lens is also caused by changes in the fine protein fibers within the eye lens, similar to the transformations we can observe when heating up a protein.

There is a lot of collagen in the lens of the eye. The proanthocyanidins contained in the cranberries influence the construction, maintenance, and degradation of the collagen positively. As a result, the cataract can be reduced by regularly supplementing the diet with PAC (commonly known as OPC = oligoproanthocyanidins). When you drink cranberry juice every day you can prevent cataracts and many other diseases. Maria Treben recommends yarrow (Achillea millefolium), Swede's herbs with eye conditions. Spirulina, chlorella, cilantro, grasses, wild herbs and other detoxifying plants can also prevent cataract as can a balanced diet with lots of fruits and vegetables, especially pumpkin and broccoli. Politics, science and health care, therefore, support the initiative committed to eating five servings of fruit and vegetables a day.

Cystitis: when the bladder is plaguing

A mild bladder infection is usually harmless and sometimes heals by itself. If, however, symptoms remain unabated for more than 48 hours, if blood is in the urine or you get a fever, you got to see a doctor. In cases of frequent recurring complaints, you better see a urologist. In addition to a contracted bladder or a lack of nerve supply, there could also be a uterine accident or a postmenopausal estrogen deficiency. Especially if no bacteria are in the urine, common cystitis could be excluded. Typical symptoms of bladder infections are frequent urination of the urine with low urine volume, unpleasant burning of the urine and pain on the pubis. As mentioned before, inflammation of the bladder is commonly caused by bacteria. These have an easy job when the natural defenses of urethra and bladder are weakened. For me, it is enough to have cold feet or sit briefly on the cool ground. Half of all women suffer from a bladder infection once in a lifetime, almost every 5th woman once a year. Next to the woman's shorter urethra than that of the man making it easier for germs to reach the bladder it is in the vicinity of the genital and anal region. E. coli bacteria can easily reach the urethra from the intestine, especially in the case of false intimate care. Also, aggressive soaps, intimate sprays or tampons can stimulate bladder infections. Sometimes the germs can even get into the kidneys causing renal cell inflammation.

Diabetes: 240 ml cranberry juice ensures constant blood glucose levels

The disease of the pancreas has to do with a lack of living food. Enzymes play a vital role in metabolism. They control and catalyze almost all biochemical reactions up to the copying of genetic information. They help in breaking down the food molecules which are then further processed by the digestive juices of the stomach, the pancreas, and the bile. Enzyme-rich fresh food helps the body's enzymes, dead food tires them and damages the pancreas. A salad before every cooked meal offers plenty of food enzymes. But before dinners, it is better to eat only avocados and papaya since other fruits and raw veggies in the eve are acid-forming and hinder digestion.

Diabetics often defy too quickly to their fate thinking they can nothing do about it. Same with my father. It seemed that he did not want to do without his daily blood glucose tests. I recommended to him Spirulina, whereupon he put two tabs into his tablet box, in the morning, two at noon, and two in the evening. I asked him, and how does the Spirulina help? He said I now only need to take a ½ insulin tablet instead of 1½. I asked, why don't you increase to 4 or 5 Spirulina tablets? Maybe then you need no other medication at all. My father, however, had always remained with his six a day.

Fernando Forato Anhê and his Canadian research team induced with an eight-week HFHS (high-fat high-sugar) diet obesity in mice. The mice treated with cranberry extract reduced weight or obesity. Liver weight and triglyceride accumulation that comes along with hepatic oxidative stress and inflammation also decreased. Above all, the insulin tolerance (2015) improved. The powerful antioxidants of cranberry help to reduce the oxidative burden associated with diabetes. Studies have shown that the supply of radical scavengers is exhausted in diabetics and persons with a very fluctuating blood glucose level. For this reason, it is essential to consume enough food with antioxidants.

Cambers and Camire from the Department of Food Science and Human Nutrition, University of Maine, examined a group of patients with diabetes. The US researchers found out that cranberry juice can reduce the side effects of diabetes and improve the quality of life of diabetics. 14 people received 6 capsules of cranberry juice powder daily for 12 weeks, the control group of 13 people received placebos. The 6 capsules correspond to 240 ml of the cranberry juice cocktail. The capsules administered to the subjects of the control group looked the same but had no active ingredients.

More than half of the patients were able to keep their blood glucose levels constant. The placebo group had higher insulin levels throughout the study. The proposal of the National Kidney Foundation to drink a glass of cranberry juice per day, however, may be too little for people with diabetes to improve their health. Since most commercial cranberry juice cocktails contain only 25-30% cranberry juice, it is likely that more concentrated

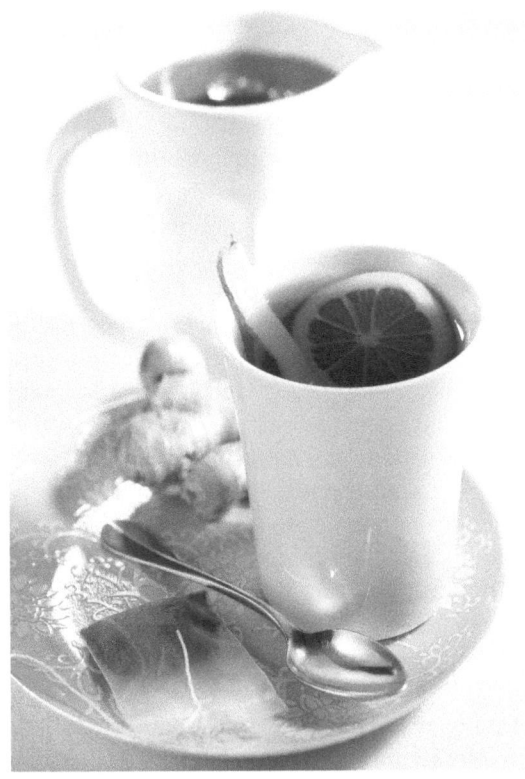

products will achieve better results. We can also stimulate the production of the body's antioxidants superoxide dismutase (SOD), catalase, and glutathione peroxidase or other enzymes thru a diet containing selenium, manganese, zinc, copper, and iron. Namely, these trace elements are required for synthesizing SOD. In addition to the phytochemicals and vitamin C, Davis and Barnard refer to other important antioxidants in cranberries for diabetics: glutathione, taurine, and alpha lipoic acid (2006). Spirulina, cinnamon and bitter melon capsules can also have a positive effect on the blood glucose. The herbalist Johann Künzle recommends a tea of 3 parts of geum alpina and golden potentila aurea, 2 parts of green dried bean peels and 1 part of blackberry and bilberry leaves: 1 heaped teaspoon per ¼ l of water, leave to draw for 3 minutes, drink 1½ -2 l daily.

Food poisoning: Cranberries protect against salmonella

Hot summers invite to barbecue and picnicking. But as the temperatures rise, the health risks are also increasing due to spoiled food.

Each year 3.000 persons die from foodborne diseases in the USA. So far, chemical preservatives have been protecting our food. However, more and more consumers are looking for natural alternatives.

Recent studies point to the unique defense strategy of cranberry against food poisoning reducing the growth of food bacteria such as salmonella and Escherichia coli. The effectiveness of cranberry has already been demonstrated in the production of cider. Apple wine is extremely susceptible to bacterial attack in an unpasteurized state.

At the annual meeting of the Institute of Food Technologists in Chicago, another study was presented. Ground meat samples, contaminated with several food bacteria, a cranberry concentrate was added. This significantly reduced the growth of salmonella.

The best thing is: We always have a spicy standard sauce in the refrigerator, which contains cranberry juice or powder. This allows us to protect salads, vegetables, fish or meat dishes from bacteria and free radicals. Simply fill a screwed glass with cold pressed oil, sea salt, cayenne pepper, mustard powder, turmeric, fresh and/or dried herbs and 2-3 teaspoons of cranberry powder. Shake, finished! See the recipe section.

Gastritis: Cranberry juice prevents the docking of Helicobacter pylori

More than 50% of the world's population harbor Helicobacter pylori in their upper gastrointestinal tract. The colonization of the stomach and its causing gastric cancer shows the complex relationship among human cells, microbes, and their environment. The inflammation of the stomach lining is caused by the insufficient response of the body to the rapidly multiplying H. pylori. This microorganism also produces a substance interfering with the metabolism of the gastric mucosa cells indirectly ensuring that too much stomach acid is produced resulting in a chronic inflammation (Amieva and Peek 2016). If we eat lots of sausage and meat, chronic gastritis can lead to stomach cancer.

Already in previous laboratory tests, a reduction of the bacteria could be detected by the proanthocyanidins (PAC) contained in the cranberries. Now, Zhang and colleagues found out in a clinical study with adults that the daily consumption of cranberry juice suppresses H. pylori infections. The authors came to the conclusion that drinking cranberry juice regularly can prevent infections by Heliobacter pylori in adults. The daily consumption of cranberry juice could be a promising new instrument in the global control of this infection (2005). So we better protect our gastric mucosa with the berry juice. Even freshly pressed organic cabbage juice can alleviate gastritis. Ginger and nutmeg in moderation as well as wild garlic and thyme, are also good for the stomach. Linseed oil, linseed, healing clay, and chamomile also have anti-inflammatory and healing properties. In times when I regularly take the oil-protein diet by Johanna Budwig, I've no stomach problems even in stressful situations. This food contains curd or cottage cheese, yellow linseed and its oil and can be seasoned as the universal mass (see recipe part).

Gingivitis: cranberries for powerful biting

This early stage of inflammation of the gums can develop when a layer of bacteria is found on the tooth. If the inflammation is not observed for a long time, extensive damage can occur around the tooth. The tooth holding apparatus, that is, the bone in which the tooth is anchored gradually breaks down.

If a gingivitis remains untreated, it can lead to chronic periodontal disease. The gum will become inflamed and shrink since no longer supported by the bone creating a gingival pocket. The tooth is slowly loosened and falls out after the destruction of its holding device or has to be pulled.

An investigation by the University of Tel Aviv concluded that a regular consumption of cranberries or the use of an oral water with Vaccinium macrocarpon reduces the risk of gum disease. For in the saliva of the participants who received cranberries, significantly fewer streptococci were found than in the saliva of the placebo group (Weiss et al., 2004).

David A Tripton and his US research colleagues studied the effect of glycated albumin and cranberry components on interleukin-6 and matrix metalloproteinase-3 production by human gingival fibroblasts. The study suggests that cranberry phenols may be useful in regulating the host response and possibly treating periodontitis in patients with poorly controlled diabetes (2016).

In addition, clove oil also disinfects the mouth and throat and acts against pathogens of various infectious diseases, including fungi, such as Candida albicans. Likewise, sage works against gum inflammation. Turmeric is generally antibacterial. See also under caries and periodontitis.

Heart disease: red card for heart diseases

Cardiovascular disorders are ruthlessly increasing as killer No. 1 in the industrial nations. According to the American Heart Association surveys the cause of death of every 2.6th US-American is a hereditary disease.

According to the Federal Statistical Office, almost every second (48%) succumb to it in 1999 in Germany. The reason is we are becoming more and more acidic because we afflict our organism with far too much acidic food. We also produce acids via stress. This sacrifices its mineral reserves to neutralize the acids. It first withdraws calcium, magnesium, and potassium from the blood vessels. The vessel walls, which have become porous by the removal of these basic minerals, must now be cemented with another substance. Our inner healer now builds up all the cholesterol available in the body and makes the vein walls tight again. In this way more and more cholesterol accumulates gradually in the blood vessels, whereby less and less blood can pass through. The blood pressure rises, the blood vessels are in danger. A ruptured cerebral vein leads to a stroke. Bursts a coronary capillary, a heart attack occurs. But recently the red berry has been showing the red card to heart disease. The American Heart Association has launched the "Go red for Women" campaign in the USA. For there, heart diseases are the main cause of death in women. One of the sponsors of the initiative is Ocean Spray, which has the largest market share of cranberry juice. Because the secondary metabolites in cranberries can contribute significantly to the health of the heart, as the following studies show:

At the University of Laval, Quebec, scientists have proven that the antioxidants in cranberries cause an increase in "good" HDL cholesterol. The ingredients of the berries improve the blood flow and contribute to the protection against heart and circulatory diseases. In 2006, Dr. Charles Couillard presented their latest research results at the annual convention of the Society of Cardiac Specialists in Calgary: HDL increased by an average of eight percent after consumption of cranberry light juice. The researcher commented: "An increase in HDL cholesterol is a sign that the arteries have been purified from the cholesterol accumulated, which is a positive effect on the heart." (Ruel et al.)

A laboratory study conducted at the William Harvey Research Institute in England showed that 1 glass of cranberry juice can be as beneficial to the heart as a glass of red wine without having the adverse effects of alcohol.

www.napsnet.com/pdf_archive/44/63304.pdf

This is good news, especially for people with an antibiotic-prone disease history as myself. I would like to do something to prevent heart and circulatory diseases. But if I regularly drink red wine, the candida multiply and soon my intestines become banquet halls. With additional stressful situations, the forming fusel alcohols cloud my clear-headedness. Since the parasites love sugar, I get the sugar-free sirup and dilute it with 3 parts of water and sweet it with Stevia.

Halima Neumann, who introduced me to the microorganism Spirulina in mid 1990th in L.A. recommends basic beverages such as 1 tbsp of Spirulina flour, 2 apples, 2 bananas, 5 figs with 2 cups of water in a blender. This delicious drink replaces any main meal. If you prefer it tart, you may appreciate the following juice: liquefy each 1 tablespoon cranberry powder and Spirulina powder, 1 cucumber, ½ onion, 1-2 tablespoons linseed oil and 1 tsp herbal salt in the mixer. By the way, if you always liquefy your salad in this way, it is digested in no time. However, salivating is important. Extra bonus: instant energy. The vital substances can already be absorbed via the oral tissue layer and brought to the cells.

Immune deficiency: bathing fun without bladder problems

Whoever drinks cranberry juice daily can prevent infectious diseases and have bathing pleasure without side effects. Cranberries contain a lot of sodium, phosphorus, potassium and vitamin C, which support the immune system defending against diseases. The even more effective ingredients in the cranberry are, the already mentioned proanthocyanidins (PAC). They affect many functions in the human body. Their antioxidant capacity is significantly higher in tests compared to vitamin C or E. They are effective radical scavengers and can prevent oxygen molecules from damaging the DNA as well as proteins and lipids.

When we drink a glass of cranberry juice every day, we strengthen our immune system. Also, laughing heartily causes the immunoglobulin A level to rise. This is a protection factor in the defense system of humans. Immunoglobulin A protects the mucous membranes of the bronchi and gastrointestinal tract from bacterial attackers.

As an active singer, I would like to point out a study by the University of Frankfurt that suggests:

Singing boosts the immune system.

In December 2004, Dr. Günter Kreutz from the Frankfurt Institute for Music Education conducted it together with the Institute for Psychology and the German Singing League. The hypothesis "Musical activities influence subjective moods and physiological processes in the autonomous nervous system" was examined at the lay choir of a Frankfurt church community. He rehearsed Mozart's Requiem for a performance. In addition to the subjective interviews, the concentrations of cortisol and immunoglobin A were also measured. The results showed significantly positive changes in the immunocompetence of the singing persons, but not in the once just listening. Franz Konz will be pleased with this study result. The singing tax and health apostle in lectures and TV shows is right after all. So, we better encourage people to get more into singing.

It would be desirable if, in the case of future health reforms, not only disease causes a negative impact on the contributions. It would be fair if singing activities in choirs and other immune boosting initiatives should be assessed. Whoever gives something to the community can also get something back.

I've been born with a weak immune system. Hence, I've given myself a kind of second immune system: In the morn, I take a few drops of colloidal silver and in the eve a few drops of colloidal gold each in a glass of water. And of course the immune boosting microalgae Spirulina platensis. Since, last year, Ursula Keim told me about her sisters, I recommend the *Green Gold* even more often: My girlfriend, a heavy smoker, is the best proof of the power of Spirulina in preventing diseases. Uschi takes the algae daily for nearly 20 years. Her two sisters are non-smoking. The elder suffers from kidney failure the younger from rheumatism. They both think it's unfair but want to know nothing of Spirulina. Or loosely based on Goethe: I hear the message well, but lack faith.

Intestinal infections: Cranberry juice prevents ulcers

Intestinal infections cause billions in healthcare costs every year. Hundreds of thousands of children die each year from infections caused by gastrointestinal viruses. An increasing number of studies show the benefit of cranberries in urinary tract infections. Therefore, Dr. Steven Lipson and colleagues from St. Francis College, Brooklyn, together with Dr. Robert Gordon of the Mount Sinai School of Medicine in New York, tested 2005 the effect of the juice on intestinal viruses in monkeys and goats. They found out that the juice prevents the clinging of the virus to red blood cells. It appears to have an effect on the replication cycle of viruses at an early stage.

https://scienceblog.com/8112/cranberry-juice-inactivates-intestinal-viruses/

However, further studies have to be carried out in humans in order to determine the usefulness of cranberry juice consumption in the reduction of viral infections of the intestine. The fresh juice of white cabbage and aloe vera also helps with inflammation of the intestine. The tea of the marigold and yarrow also works favorably on the intestine as does the Swedish herbs.

Irritable bladder: the bladder as a mirror of the psyche

We experience physical discomfort in response to psychosocial stress. The physical sensation makes our feelings noticeable: blushing, butterflies in the belly, goose bumps, heart palpitations, soft knees. The complaints seem to be physical. But they are not. Because the emotional stress leads to a physical reaction: we feel butterflies in the abdomen, our hairs are resisting, we get cold feet, the blood is up, it gets to us or puts pressure on the bladder. Or we are scared.

The irritable bladder is not a typical phenomenon of aging and a natural consequence of births but a common disease. Many sufferers hide behind a wall of silence and shame. Some people's complaints are so pronounced that they hardly dare to go public. The bladder irritates in all age groups, in women more frequently than in men. In Germany, about six million persons are affected by various forms of urinary incontinence. There are no exact numbers for the irritable bladder. It is often associated with urinary tract infection (UTI) or uterine disease. However, many other factors trigger an increased urge to urinate, especially tensions and anxiety.

The exact causes of the irritable bladder are not known. A sudden urge to urinate occurs when the bladder muscle cramps. If this happens because the nerves report a false "filling state" to the brain or it is a wrongly learned habit is unclear. The urge to urinate usually occur in certain situations, for example, in the case of mental strain or cold feet. However, the fear of renewed sudden urination can cause the symptoms to increase in intensity and occur in more and more situations. Excessive consumption of alcohol, coffee or nicotine can also worsen the symptoms. Sometimes they are so massive that a normal life is impossible because of the constant visits to the toilets. The amount of urine emitted is only very small. Occasionally, there is also a burning sensation when passing urine.

An infection of the urinary tract in which bacteria are usually detected in the urine can cause symptoms similar to those of the irritable bladder. An UTI can be prevented with cranberry juice. In women, a prolapse of the uterus, in men a prostate disease has to be ruled out. It is also important to recognize the situations leading to urinary urge.

Here a micturition diary can be helpful. When you write down what you have eaten and drunk, or when and in what situation you need to go to the toilet, you can possibly rule out an organic status. After some time, you will recognize certain trigger patterns.

The bladder is the mirror of the psyche. It is nervously supplied by the vegetative nervous system. Therefore, not only pulse and sweat production increase during excitement. Also, the visits to the toilets are more frequent. Just think of examinations, introductory talks, presentations when most women and men suffer from an overactive bladder. Sometimes you do not realize that you are under psychological pressure. Any pressure demands to let go and relax. If this is not achieved psychologically you must allow it physically. An anxiety-inducing experience causes an upset bowel. That's why it is said: It scared the shit out of me. During the Northridge earthquake in California, I realized this. We lived only about 4 miles from the epicenter. Also before a lecture, I have to empty the bladder pushing the psychological pressure into the bladder and feeling here as physical pressure. This pressure detour makes it clear how painful it can be if you do not let go and how liberating it is when you do.

The therapy of an irritable bladder seems as solving a puzzle. If stress is the cause, the immune-boosting cranberry is helpful in any case. Because stress weakens our inner healer the most. Often, the stimulus can be brought under control by medication, psychotherapy or relaxation techniques and continence training. Sometimes acupuncture, acupressure, and biofeedback also, the homeopathic medicines Pulsatilla or Dulcamara can help. Lady's mantle tea is supposed to strengthen the musculature. See also chapter How much juice does the bladder boost?
www.medicinenet.com/urinary_tract_infection/article.htm

Kidney stones: cranberry for prevention

My father could have told you a thing or two about the torments of hell, which caused a kidney stone sticking in the urinary tract. By contrast, labor should be a leisurely Sunday stroll. The number of new cases worldwide is increasing. Above all, more and more women suffer from nephrolithiasis with increasing age. Kidney stones are associated with a chronic renal disease. Causes are usually an acidic diet and stress. As is known, drugs such as protease inhibitors, antibiotics, and some diuretics increase the risk of some types of kidney stones. It is better to prevent the formation of kidney stones with a suitable supply of nutrients. You can alkalize the urine by consuming a diet high in fruits, vegetables, salads and basic mineral water. To avoid calcium phosphate and struvite stones, the urine should be acidified; cranberry juice can lower the pH of the urine. Researchers at the University of California School of Medicine in San Francisco (Frassetto and Kohlstadt 2011) proved it. Lemons also have a stone-inhibiting effect: 1 lemon in 1 liter of water; sweetened with stevia or honey.

Macular degeneration: lutein and zeaxanthin guard against

Free radicals associate with age-related disease. As the retina of the eye consumes a lot of oxygen, it is particularly susceptible to oxidative stress. It also contains large quantities of polyunsaturated fatty acids and is always exposed to light. The two carotenoids lutein and zeaxanthin in cranberry appear to play an important role in the retina of the eye. For, in the macula lutea of the eye only the carotenoids lutein and zeaxanthin occur. The macula lutea is responsible for detail recognition at the center of the visual field. It is assumed that a lack of lutein and zeaxanthin in this part of the retina leads to ADM. This age-related degeneration of the macula is the main cause of age blindness in the industrialized countries. The yellow-orange xanthophyll lutein contained in cranberries is next to the beta-carotene the most widespread carotenoid. Researchers from around the world confirm the correlation between AMD and low carotenoid concentrations. The visual acuity increased in a study, especially in blue-eyed persons. (Dagnelie, 2000). Bone and his team were able to show in the living and the deceased: AMD patients show a significantly lower lutein and zeaxanthin concentration in the macula (Bone et al, 2000, 2001).

In a recent study, Taiwanese researchers focused on the effect of cranberry juice (CJ) on blue light imitating the human retinal pigment epithelium (ARPE-19) cells imitating age-related macular degeneration (AMD). They found that the condensed tannin in cranberry juice showed a greater rinsing effect and better repairability (increased cell viability) implying that a better radical scavenging activity to effectively protect the ARPE-19 cells thus stopping the progress of the AMD (Chang et al., 2017).

Therefore it is advisable to start early with the regular consumption of cranberry products to prevent age blindness.

Pancreas: when parasitic fungi are plaguing

A variety of infectious factors is related to acute pancreatitis. Pathologic or radiologic detection of pancreatitis associated with a well-documented infection is reported with viruses, bacteria, fungi, and parasites.

In 1968, Swartz and Medrek established the antifungal effects of the cranberry juice in the Department of Dermatology and Bacteriology of the Massachusetts General Hospital in Boston. The in vitro study investigated eight species of fungi. Seven showed the antifungal action of the berry juice. Only the Candida albicans remained unmoved by the cranberry. The sugar content of the juice is usually high and sugar is the favorite food of this invasive yeast fungus. In a newer study, French scientists added a dry commercial extract of cranberry fruit (Vaccinium macrocarpon Aiton) to the culture medium, displaying a significant anti-adhesion activity against Candida (Girardot 2014). With a yeast infection, we better use cranberry sirup or powder and make our own juice or find brands sweetened with Stevia or other natural sugar-free sweetener.

Periodontitis: Cranberries prevent bacteria from adhering to teeth

Aside from caries periodontosis is the most frequent cause of teeth loss. Both diseases are caused by bacteria in the dental plaque. A natural diet with plenty of raw food and regular care with the removal of the dental plaque on teeth and gums is the best protection against caries, periodontal disease, and tooth loss. Permanent stress or test anxiety can severely reduce the immune defense of the body and trigger a gum inflammation. As a result of the reduced immune defense, the concentration of the protective factor immunoglobulin A decreases in the saliva. Therefore, the harmful bacteria in the mouth have an easy play, according to the Düsseldorf periodontist and chairman of the International Academy for Dental Reconstruction, Hans-Dieter John.

www.mednews.blogg.de

Periodontitis increases the risk of cardiovascular disease, diabetes, and chronic respiratory disease. Conversely, certain diseases can affect oral health. For example, diabetics, dialysis patients, transplant patients, and people with hypertension are at risk since they usually take different drugs. Certain medicines can also lead to changes in the blood pressure of the gums, which promote increased plaque accumulation and the development of gum disease (gingivitis).

As early as 1998 a study by the University of Tel Aviv indicated that certain compounds in the cranberry prevent the attachment of various domestic bacteria in the mouth, of bacteria on teeth and other bacteria. This is apparently the same mechanism that prevents the docking also responsible for the health of the urinary tract (Weiss et al.).

Plaque/bleeding gums: cranberry juice for prevention

Dental plaque adheres as a film almost invisible to the human eye on the tooth surface. For daily care, remove it best after breakfast and before going to bed with floss, a toothbrush and toothpaste minimizing the risk of millions of bacteria remaining on the tooth or the gumline. Otherwise, inflammation of the adjacent gingival area may develop, swell up, become red leading to gum bleeding. Since no pain occurs bleeding is an alarm signal, which is very serious. If this inflammation persists for an extended period, gingivitis develops. See also under gingivitis, caries, and periodontitis.

Since cranberries can prevent bacteria from sticking on, it is advisable to drink a glass of sugar-free cranberry juice every morning and evening. We can also prepare mouthwash with the acidic fruit. I make colloidal silver with 99,99 % silver rods and mix this silver water half with cranberry sirup from the health food store.

Poor digestion: The bitter substances of the cranberry stimulate gastric juices

As we can easily find out when biting into the fruit, cranberries contain bitters. These act as a natural eating control and reduce the appetite for sweets. They also stimulate the production of the digestive juices necessary for the breakdown of the food: the stomach pours out more hydrochloric acid and pepsin. On the way to the small intestine, the liver adds enzymes (biliary salts and acids), which further break down the food pulp. The pancreas enhances the enzymes amylase, trypsin and lipase. This way, the organism pours out more food-cleaving enzymes allowing it to process nutrients better and faster. Standing for better digestion and particularly tempting less fat over the frame.

Rheumatoid arthritis (RA): Can crippling form back?

Yes, absolutely I know it from my girlfriend Carole. She had already deformed finger joints. How did she get rid of this inflammatory foci? Carole had strictly adhered to the Eat Right for Your Blood Type Diet (D'Adamo and Whitney: 4 Blood Groups - Four Strategies for a Healthy Life). Heavy-heartedly she eliminated red meat. With that, she got rid of all her deformed knuckles. This confirms the experience of a fellow travel companion. Mike is always miraculously healed from his rheumatism overwintering in Morocco. He had discovered that it was the pork. But at home, he can not stay away from the fat sausages and the ham.

Studies indicate that the autoimmune disease is triggered by urinary tract infections with Proteus bacteria. Ebringer and Rashid of Kings College, London, proceeded from the following considerations: Chronic deforming polyarthritis occurs particularly in middle-aged and older women. The extensive various microbial, immunological and molecular studies from all over the world show: There is a strong connection between Proteus mirabilis microbes and rheumatoid arthritis (RA). These rod bacteria belong to the Enterobacteriaceae family. These bacteria of the intestinal tract include E. coli, shigella, and salmonella. The researchers assume that urine infections with Proteus are the main trigger factors of the RA. The presence of molecular mimicry and cross-reacting between these bacteria and tissue antigens affected by RA still support the ongoing disease process through the production of cell-pathological autoantibodies (2006). Patients with this disease could particularly benefit in the early stages of Proteus antibacterial agents, a vegetarian diet, plenty of water and cranberry juice. Perhaps in this way, we will soon be able to contain further autoimmune diseases and many other health problems. Halima Neumann advises in her book *Stop der Azidose, Allergien und Haarausfall* for base excess diet. In order to promote healing gout and rheumatism, she recommends consuming twice a day half a pound of celery root (also as juice).

Salmonellosis: healthy despite rotten meat

If you do not want to eliminate animal products, you will have to reckon with salmonella infections. But perhaps we can prevent food poisoning by regular cranberry consumption.

Riitta Puggupponen-Pimia and her colleagues attribute selected phenolic components of cranberry and some other red and blue berries the following effects: They inhibit the growth of pathogens such as salmonella and staphylococci in the gastrointestinal tract. The Finnish researchers do not exclude that the antimicrobial activity of the berries can also be associated with their anti-adhesion effect. They assume that antimicrobial berry components will find many uses as a natural protection against microorganisms in the food industry as well as in medicine (2005).

It gives us reason to hope that in the future even fast-food consumers will consume at least berry ingredients if they do without the whole vital fuel bombs.

Stomach ulcer: Cranberry juice dispels *Helicobacter*

Good news for tourists: 2 glasses of cranberry juice daily can protect the stomach from bacterial infection and ulcers. In China, 80% of all gastric ulcers are caused by Helicobacter pylori bacteria, while in North America and Central Europe it is 30%. The Berlin Robert Koch Institute has found a prevalence rate of 40% among the German population. Researchers at the Peking University in cooperation with colleagues from the UCLA in California investigated: 2 glasses of cranberry juice daily can protect the stomach from bacterial infection and ulcers. In the cranberry group, the bacteria were suppressed three times more frequently than in the control group. This clinical study published in the March 2005 edition of the medical specialist Helicobacter suggests: Cranberry fruit juice drink (Cranberry Classic) is effective against the bacteria that most frequently cause gastric ulcers.

The daily consumption of cranberry juice could thus help to reduce the number of 160,000 patients treated annually in Germany for stomach ulcers. The latter occur when the Heliobacter pylori bacteria succeed in introducing themselves into the protective mucous membranes of the gastric walls, and to ignite them.

The folk medicine knows yet another plant, which acts against gastric trouble: the thyme.

Stroke: Cranberry's polyphenols prevent brain attacks

Young people can already have a heart attack. The genetic metabolic Fabry disease is one of the causes. Neurologists from Rostock found a specific enzyme missing in the metabolism (Rolfs et al., 2005). The enzyme agalactosidase should degrade a certain fatty substance which is instead deposited in the most diverse cell types such as in the heart muscle and renal cells. Sometimes the disease is diagnosed only when the kidneys are already chronically damaged happening to my father. He had a fat and weak heart as well as constant problems with the kidneys and died of a cerebral hemorrhage.

The OPC or PAC in cranberries counting to the polyphenols inhibit the activity of platelets. If the platelets stick together, blood clots may develop damaging the blood vessels and risk an increase in cardiovascular diseases. In the recipe section, you'll find a cranberry chocolate. With its double-high polyphenol content, it can reduce the risk pleasantly. Phenols also reduce the harmful LDL cholesterol. This can react in the body with oxygen. Oxidized LDL cholesterol is considered to be a contributory cause of arteriosclerosis, which is known to induce myocardial infarction and stroke. Researchers have found that cranberries and cocoa can significantly reduce this reaction. See also the next chapter.

Thrombosis: prophylaxes instead of support stockings.

People who like my mother take Marcumar must always pay attention to what they eat. Often, the most healthy vegetable or fruit variety they are not allowed to eat. Many of these patients may not need any anticoagulant if they'd regularly exercise, drink cranberry juice, use garlic as well as eat lots of fruits and vegetables. Some of our contemporaries do not care about prevention. You can get this information when you visit the forums Thrombosis-DVT-Anxiety or Marcumar forever. Already 22-year-olds participate in the chat and ask: Must I take the stuff forever? Is it possible to dispense completely with a corresponding diet? Some of the young commuting women smoke, take the birth control pill and barely exercise.

So, if you do not want to wear the anti-sex stockings, better take quick preventive action: After leaving the forum, I had a strange feeling in the left lower leg. So be careful! Hypochondriacs should better avoid the public discourse. I immediately made a headstand and dissolved a tablespoon of cranberry powder in my green tea and cut two cloves of garlic into my vegetable dish.

I have not found a convincing study proving that cranberry juice leads to more severe bleeding when drinking with anticoagulants. However, after a patient had postoperative hemorrhages drinking cranberry juice in conjunction with taking blood coagulation inhibitors, Grant noted that patients taking warfarin (anticoagulant) should limit their cranberry juice consumption (2004). The Rindone and Murphy report does not convince me either. It is based on the experience of a single patient having developed a strong hemorrhage after his fixed dose of warfarin. This happened shortly after he had started with the daily consumption of cranberry juice. No other reason for the pronounced hypothrombinemia (coagulation disorder) could be identified. Therefore, the researchers assume a definite link between cranberry juice and warfarin.

It would be much more interesting to examine whether persons taking Marcumar could change to Ibuprofen with daily cranberry juice or cranberry preparations or to acetylsalicylic acid (ASA) or Aspirin®. The constant blood tests are annoying for the patients; they also weigh the cash registers. Of the possible long-term effects of the coagulation inhibitors for once leaving aside.

The brother of a friend took Marcumar without having the prothrombin values checked regularly. When the man in his mid-forties got very red toes, he dropped the medication. The abnormal bleeding went back immediately. Since his tablets were a problem with high blood pressure, he took garlic pills that kept his blood pressure constant. We have now advised him to test the cranberry capsules, especially since Ferry suffers from an autoimmune disease and the Vaccinium macrocarpon also arouses hope here (see chapter Rheumatoid Arthritis (RA): Can crippling form back?). Would it not be a blessing (except, of course, for the disease industry), if the power berry could also cure these civilization diseases?

On August 30, 2006, I went with my mother to her health practitioner in Fürth. I asked him if my mother was allowed to have cranberries. Raimon Schacker said: "Yes, she can eat them. Although the cranberry changes the consistency of the blood, it does not dilute it." Amazed by this spontaneous feedback, I looked at him open-mouthed. He must have understood this as if I did not understand because he clasped his fingers and explained: "The protein molecules are linked together in such a way (he raised his hands). The cranberry stretches these fiber connections (he stretched his fingers and moved them apart slowly). The molecules are separated. The blood is changed consistently, but not in the coagulation phase. I was baffled. Is this tanned muscular man a sort of Edgar Cayce? The famous sleeping prophet, through channeling, was always able to pass on the right behavioral remedies to his visitors seeking for health advice. Mr. Schacker looking into his patient's eyes also pattering everything he sees at incredible speed, his facial expressions and gestures are also changing. His polished Buddha-head moves sometimes abruptly. Everything sounds very plausible, very understandable. When I asked him if he receives messages from a "higher level" he only smiled mysteriously moving his head like an Indian. As if to say, maybe I am the reincarnation of the trance healer of Virginia Beach.

Whether you believe what the health expert has said about the cranberry or not, you can test it on your own if you need to take an anticoagulant. When others tell you their experiences, it does not have to be the same for you. Every organism reacts differently. When we learn to listen and to interpret our body, we also know how to be healed and to live a long, healthy life.

Urinary tract infections: Belly shows can end painfully

When the sun blares down, we spend the days at the lake or swimming pool and scarcely notice whether the bikini is wet or not. If we feel ill at ease afterward, an inflammation of the urethra is often the cause of the pain.

Cranberry juice has long been appreciated for its beneficial effect in preventing urinary tract disorders. In March 1994, researchers from the Harvard Medical School conducted the first controlled and broad clinical trial. It was to prove that the regular consumption of *Cranberry Juice Cocktail* significantly reduced the presence of bacteria in the urinary tract. Avorn and colleagues found that the effect is not due to a stronger acidity in the urine. The urine of the cranberry juice drinkers was by no means more acidic than those of persons who took a placebo drink without cranberries. The researchers suspected that cranberry contains something specific that prevents bacteria from adhering to the urinary tract area. This study was carried out with 153 women with an average age of 78 years. They drank daily 300 ml of the above-mentioned drink with a cranberry juice content of 27 percent. Their findings suggest:

Using a cranberry beverage reduces the frequency of bacteriuria with pyuria (pus in the urine) in older women (1994).

In a small double-blind clinical study (when physicians and patients do not know who gets what substance), researchers at Weber State University found out that sexually active women aged 18 to 45 who received a dietary food supplement over a period of 6 months of spray-dried cranberry juice were significantly less likely to have urinary tract infections than women who took a placebo (Walker et al., 1997).

But it was only Amy Howell and her colleagues coming to the conclusion that the substances contained in cranberry juice Vaccinium proanthocyanidins are responsible for the health-promoting effect in the area of the urinary tract (1998). The scientific team at Rutgers University identified the active substances responsible for the health of the urinary tract: the proanthocyanidins (PAC) or condensed tannins. These compounds crucial for cranberry's anti-adhesion effect, are characterized by a special biochemical compound (A-type PAC). This makes them different from the PAC in green tea or chocolate. The latter, differently structured PAC, do not exhibit this particular anti-adhesive property. Three years later, researchers at Rutgers University found out that the cranberry proanthocyanidins are absorbed by the body. This suggests that the proanthocyanidins once taken and entering the bloodstream become available at other body sites. Thus, they can exert the anti-adhesion and/or antioxidant effect (Howell et al., 2001).

Medical examinations at the University of Oulu, Finland, showed that the consumption of cranberry fruit juice could reduce the recurrence of urinary tract infections in the women under investigation by as much as 50 percent. Previous studies have already linked cranberry to the reduction of urinary tract infections. These results further support the preventive function of cranberry in this type of infection (Kontiokari et al., 2001). In a later study, the Finnish researchers confirm the reduced likelihood of UTI by using fresh berry juices. They state that dietary advice may be a first step towards the prevention of urinary tract infections (2003).

In 2002 Lynn Stothers examined 150 sexually active women between 21 and 72 randomly divided into three prophylaxis groups for one year: placebo juice plus placebo tablets, cranberry juice plus placebo tablets and placebo juice plus cranberry tablets. The participants took the tablets twice daily and drank the juice (250 ml) three times a day. Both preventive measures significantly reduced the number of patients who had at least one urinary tract infection in the study year (18 and 20% versus 32%, respectively). The patients had to take fewer antibiotics, required fewer pantyliners and were less likely to miss work. The savings due to prevention were greatest in patients with more than two symptomatic UTIs (with three days of antibiotic therapy) and more than two sick leave days in patients who needed urge incontinence pads. The cranberry tablets provided the most cost-effective prevention of urinary tract infections.

James Greenberg, a gynecologist at the Women's Hospital in Boston, USA, wanted to know whether this effect could be demonstrated when taking dried cranberries. His team conducted a small pilot study with five women suffering from urinary tract infection. Their urine was examined after taking Ocean Spray Craisins (dried, naturally flavored and sweetened cranberries). The analysis showed the anti-stick activity increasing by 50% meaning that even dried cranberries can make life difficult for bacteria.

The unique structure of the proanthocyanidins found in cranberries is responsible for the anti-infective properties. As a result, certain particularly virulent uropathogenic E-coli bacteria can no longer dock on the walls of the urinary tract. These strains, equipped with trapping arms, are easily rinsed from the body without causing any damage. The pilot study suggests that not only the cranberry juice but also other forms of the fruit have these anti-infective properties.

Halima Neumann recommends celery juice cures for all kinds of bladder trouble. For kidney and bladder diseases she advises aloe vera essence and barley or wheat grass juice because these have a particularly healing and analgesic effect.

The miraculous transformation of rods into spheres

Scientists have now discovered the unique effect of the cranberry juice: inhibiting the adhesion of certain Coli bacteria. The proanthocyanidins (PAC) or condensed tannins in cranberries were recognized as accountable ingredients. How are these microbes prevented from docking in the urinary tract and causing infections? The PAC attack the rod bacteria and transform them into spherical structures. In addition, they also balk the communication between microbes destroying the small hooks bacteria use to stick onto the bladder wall. Before the germs can multiply and trigger an inflammation, they are flushed out. The infection preventing effect depends on the property of certain ingredients to prevent the formation of biofilm. Also, persons who drink cranberry juice excrete inflammatory-inhibiting salicylic acid.

http://en.wikipedia.org/wiki/Cranberry

However, when the E. coli bacteria have first penetrated into the mucous membranes of the urinary tract, they cause constant urge to urinate and burning during passing water. The doctor will then prescribe antibiotics to counter the risk of renal insufficiency. I only work with natural antibiotics such as colloidal silver, grapefruit seed extract, sometimes also 30% Hydrogen peroxide (H_2O_2).

Prevention with the redskin is essential

The cranberry can not kill the pathogens actively. Therefore, they also help little in an existing infection. This was confirmed by two persons suffering from cystitis, who could not report any success in cranberry during an acute infection. But against the risks of a new infection, we can prevent with cranberry juice (morning and evening 75 ml of sirup or 200 ml of cranberry juice mixtures). Because the proanthocyanidins (PAC) of the American cranberry prevent the docking of the Escherichia coli bacteria on the urinary tract through the anti-adhesion mechanism already found in May 1984 by US researchers: 0.45 l *Cranberry Juice Cocktail* significantly limit the adhesion of bacteria of the group E. coli in the test persons. Since these are the cause of urinary tract infections in 80 to 90 percent of the cases, we can maintain the urinary tract healthy through the unique cranberry.

Researchers at the University of Tel Aviv in 1991 confirmed the anti-adhesion effect of cranberry juice. They tried to identify the substances in the berries that are responsible for this process. Ofek and colleagues came to the conclusion that a combination of substances of unknown nature prevents E. coli bacteria from adhering to the bladder wall. The juices of oranges, pineapples, mangoes, guavas and grapefruits, however, did not show this anti-adhesion effect.

What else can we do for the bladder?

Usually, the following measures are recommended to reduce the risk of urinary tract infection: drink at least 30 ml of water per kg of body weight daily. Herbal remedies or tea made from goldenrod can alleviate symptoms. Goldenrod can reduce the frequency of passing water. Pumpkin seeds have a similar effect as well as teas made from bearberry leaves or restharrow. Bearberry leaf preparations (tea, extract, capsules) can not only disinfect the urinary tract.

Its active substance arbutin or hydroquinone are also carcinogenic and can damage the liver. Therefore they should be taken only a few times a year.

The nettle, birch, horsetail and juniper stimulate the kidney to produce urine. While passing urine, it is important to empty the bladder completely and sit straight. Bent-over sitting on the toilet prevents total emptying of the bladder. Warm clothing on the abdomen protects against bladder infections.

The drinking of cranberry juice before and the passing urine immediately after sexual intercourse prevents the adhesion of bacteria and rinses the urethra. It is important to avoid dampness and cold. Also, beware of hot spices, black tea, coffee, and alcohol. Contradictory instructions may cause uncertainty: avoiding sour foods or taking baking soda to keep the urine alkaline. On the other hand, the sour cranberry juice helps demonstrably. It is best to try what is good for you. Also, it may change. Nothing remains as it is: neither in the universe nor in the smallest microorganism. The more complicated our life is, the more it eats our vitality. Thus, bladder trouble can also be due to lack of nerve supply. Therefore it is not often enough to avoid stress and constant tension. Because tense bladder walls reduce mucus production increasing the risk of bacteria adhering in the bladder region. This is why daily breathing exercises, yoga, or autogenic training should be a daily regimen.

Can the cranberry turn the clock back?

This at least suggests the study Zhu and his colleagues conducted at the National Institute on Aging in Baltimore. They investigated the effects of long-term cranberry consumption on age-related changes in endocrine pancreas in 344 male fishermen rats. The researchers supplemented the normal rodent chow with 2% cranberry powder. Both groups showed an age-related decline in basal plasma insulin concentrations but this age-related decline was delayed by cranberry (2011).

I experienced with cranberries an energy boost needing less sleep and having more endurance. From my experience and taking into account the many effects of the red miracle fruit, confirmed by international scientific investigations, the idea came to me cranberry could be the Methuselah fruit par excellence. Could it be that it helps to youthful vigor again? After all, it contains the strongest antioxidants ever found in a fruit and is proven to help with age-related diseases such as arteriosclerosis and macular degeneration of the retina (ADM).

In the search for answers, I then found cases of high age documented by Guinness World Records. This was created with the help of the Gerontology Research Group of the University of California. It is a global database of people aged 100 and over. http://www.grg.org/

I noticed:

Of the documented oldest 30 women in the world, 14 come from North America! There were 5 British, 4 Japanese, 3 French: then only inhabitants of individual states. In Great

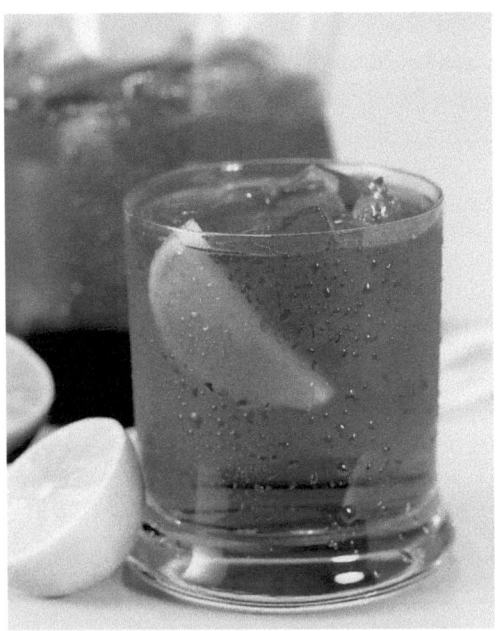

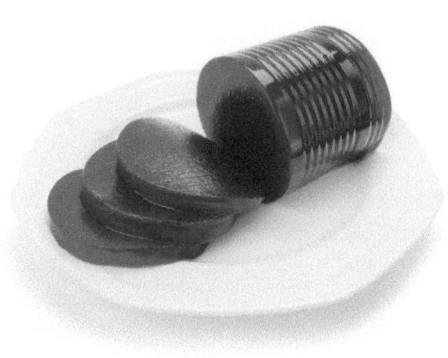

That North Americans eat cranberries in the cold season is known. Also, with bladder problems they regularly drink cranberry juice to prevent new infections for its healing effect is known by every child in America. I was talking to my elderly friend who lived in the US for fifty years. Almost all her friends and acquaintances drink or drank the juice. I urged her also back in Berlin to drink cranberry juice regularly. She said, in L. A. I always had several ½ gallon bottles in the house. They were cheap there. I said, yes but it is only a mixture with a quarter of a liter of pure cranberry juice.

If you buy 1 l of sirup, divide it into ¼ l bottles you can make 4 liters for about €8. If you sweeten the juice with stevia you get a better quality. Three of the little bottles you pack into the freezer, the rest in the large bottle you fill up with water.

Britain and France, the healing effects of cranberry are known and used. Japanese people enjoy the longest life expectancy of all citizens of the industry. But though Japan has the same amount of inhabitants as the UK and French together they have only half of the amount of Methuselah. All persons with biblical age were assigned to their country of birth. Many of them have emigrated to North America! Can it really have been due to the cranberries that these people have grown so old? You may now say this is pure speculation. But if you read the scientific studies in the chapter DISEASE PREVENTION AND HEALING FROM A-Z and also about the secondary metabolites, you may share my enthusiasm.

Now we do not all need to move to the Yankees to extend our life expectancy. Let's try it every day with a glass of cranberry juice growing in the USA and Canada. Let's take the chance to do something good for our health. By the way, on the 27th of August 2006, the day when I discovered the list for the first time, Maria Esther Capovilla died at the age of 116. A month later she would have been 117. Today there are other individuals leading the list as you can see by using the link below.

This filling-up/infusion I had to explain to Hilde several times. I thought that had to do with her diet and the lack of exercise. Recently I had a few days with her in Berlin. She ate little fresh food. I then called my mother, who was almost the same age, to test her mental flexibility. When I began to explain to her the three little bottles, she took my word off and said, and the rest I dilute with water. My mother ate fruits every morning and had 6 or 7 berry bushes in the garden. She was very active.

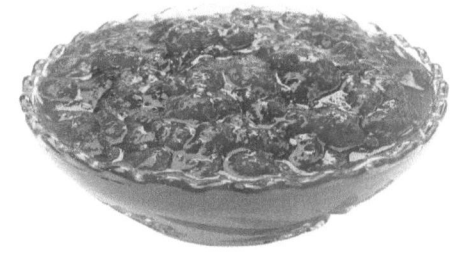

V. PROGRESS REPORTS: EXPERIENCE AND PERCEPTION

This chapter is a bit short. I hope, however, I will get more information for the next edition. Why do many people talk about their bladder problems only with the hand over their mouth:? Perhaps because most of those having no bladder problems associate with it only organ weakness and uncontrolled urination. We usually have the pictures of seniors in mind, which make advertising for Pampers. And who wants to be reminded of a possible future reality?

Distress during coitus

A few years ago, I'd been experiencing pain during the world's most beautiful incidental event. And although I always empty the bladder before, I suffered from a painful urge to urinate as if something was blocking. I ventured the rare visit to the family doctor, especially since my blood had not been tested for a long time. When I picked up the results, the doctor said, if I hadn't a slight under-function of the thyroid gland, I could go on an exhibition with my blood count. I subsequently took seaweed preparations for the thyroid and went to the internist. Also, nothing wrong. The urine samples were negative. So after thirty years I even dared to go to the gynecologist. He did not find anything wrong. I asked, "What could be this resistance connected with pain?" Shrugging his shoulders, the doctor recommended creams for sex. As if I had not already had thought of it myself. After consulting three doctors, I had enough of medical advice for the next ten years. If I had listened to my inner voice, I would probably have known that my problems are connected with tensions and anxiety. Because on holidays my bladder hardly irritates and at night it leaves me also in peace. Since then, I regularly consume cranberry juice and eat the creations listed in the recipe section: the problems seem to be history.

Distress after coitus

M. K. received a bladder infection each time after sexual intercourse with severe pain. I brought cranberry to her attention. She then took a cranberry capsule from the pharmacy in the morning, and in the evening, and drank a glass of diluted cranberry sirup from the health food store each time after lovemaking. The next morning she drank another glass and in the evening once again. Lo and behold, until now she had no bladder infections. However, when she neglects the water drinking during the day, she can still feel her bladder. Drinking a lot of water and cranberry juice quickly, she is symptom-free a few hours later.

Hardening - the Barefoot of Beerfelden

On June 22, 2006, I gazed at a middle-aged woman. I was standing at the supermarket in the vegetable section when she passed me: barefoot on the stone floor! I said, laughing, "You've never had anything to do with the bladder?" No, she said. I am used to it. I always walk barefoot. But you have to start very slowly, with a minute. I have exaggerated it first. I became quite sick.

She is right. At times I also toughened up with cold water. Only I'm weak at regularity. Only with yoga, I'm resolute. After all, the woman from Beerfelden motivated me to start again with cold rubbings. Unfortunately, she did not report to me. I gave her my flyer hoping she'd write a comment on my website. You can also do this if you want to contribute to health, environment, animal protection, and counseling:
www.marianne-e-meyer.com

Cranberry mobilizes memory capacity

By the way, I noticed that my memory capacity had back its old freshness by the regular consumption of the cranberry. Before, I had problems with my short-term memory. I also do not need so much sleep, work physically in the household and garden more than before, and still write four or five books a year. So if you have problems with the concentration and memory retention skills, try the cranberry. In any case, you are doing something good for you. If it does not help your memory, it strengthens your immune system and your cardiovascular system.

Painful bladder as blown away

R. S. suffered from a painful urge to urinate without producing much urine. I gave her some bags of cranberry powder (Urovit®) for testing. She was totally surprised at the effect and immediately got a big pack. Meanwhile, she had once again a starting bladder infection. She then increased the dose to three times a day and drunk a lot of water. In the evening everything was okay again.

Short story for the coincidence album

We've all buried a treasure somewhere that we guard more or less. My treasure chest is full of so-called coincidences. When I moved to California with my husband 30 years ago, they magnified in rapid succession. Therefore, I considered it my task to publish my coincidental album. If you are not afraid of ghost stories, you can read them in my book *FAMILY CODE*.

For my choir practice after the summer break 2006, I had printed the study of the Frankfurt Institute for Music Education. I wanted to inform the choir members that they are strengthening their immune system by actively singing. But there were so many music performances to discuss, that I did not get to do it. After the chorus, Friedel asked, does one of you go to the Schwarz? I was not sure and said to win time, Jessica (the prominent acting daughter of the Rathausbräu owner) is now the first smoker in the state, at least the picture gallery in the *Spiegel* mag began with her. Since the tavern is on my way, I thought I'd decide while walking. Suddenly I remembered the pleasing study result. As in a trance, I crumbled the sheet out of my pocket when I heard voices behind me. Two of the female choir members reached me. One looked over my shoulder and called in surprise: Cranberry! Do you know the cranberry? I said yes, I am writing a book about it. Gabriele Pfeiffer-Junischke said. Oh, then I can tell you a story: I was at the doctor because I had blood in the urine. He gave me an antibiotic. On the next examination, there was still as much blood in the urine. He said, drink some cranberry juice. On the way to the health food store, I roamed over a remnants market. And what did my delighted eyes see on the shelf? A single glass of cranberries, whole fruits in juice. I cleaned out the whole glass. And on the next day, the urine was clear.

I dare to read the thoughts of some of my readers: That can be a coincidence. Perhaps even without the cranberries, no blood would have been in the urine. Sure it can be. But what keeps us from giving the power berry a chance? Especially if the antibiotics do not help. I always say: our experience is what creates knowledge. And that is true science.

After a few days a lot of energy and super coagulation test

At the beginning of September 2006, I brought my mother the cranberry powder. She had been given the green light by her health practitioner. Despite taking Marcumar, she was able to eat the blood-thinning berry. She'd been drinking two glasses of juice a day. On September 11, she could not sleep. Usually, she drinks a glass of milk and goes back to bed. But this time she stayed in the kitchen at two o'clock, clearing all the cabinets and wiping all the floors. Apart from the energy rise, she'd not noticed anything yet. She said it could also be the Lapacho tea, she'd been drinking again. Lapacho is also anti-inflammatory, works against cancer and acts against candida yeast fungus. I asked, have you ever had such energy thrusts from the tea cleaning at night? I think it would be good to have a health logbook. Then we could look up the reactions to certain remedies later.

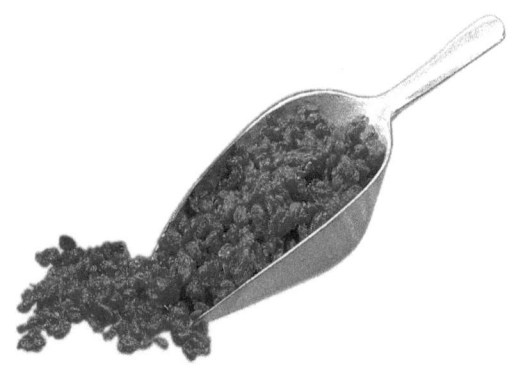

A few days later, my mother invited us to a plum cake and told us about her visit to the doctor the day before. For the first time in the 5 or 6 years that she needs to take marcumar, the prothrombin time (PT) allowed her to take fewer tablets until the next test. This test is a laboratory parameter of the functional performance of the extrinsic system of blood clotting. The Prothrombin time builds the basis for monitoring oral vitamin K antagonists such as marcumar, warfarin, and phenindione.

How much juice does the bladder boost?

Sometimes I have the impression that my bladder is taking on a life of itself. If I only come near a toilet, it suddenly starts to press. But if I'm underway, make a bike ride or have an interesting conversation it seems to completely switch off.

If my bladder annoys again, I get cranberry sirup from the health food store. In the morning and in the evening a glass of 70 ml is sufficient to prevent urinary tract infections. If you prefer the cocktail mixed with water or other cranberry juices you need at least 200 ml. As mentioned earlier,

cranberries contain condensed tannins hindering bacteria from adhering to the urinary tract cells for up to ten hours preventing infections.

However, bacteria were never found in my urine. Therefore, as the main cause of my bladder problems, I suspect stress and/or cold feet or chilly seating surfaces. For during the day the urine urges up to ten times. But if I sleep under a warm blanket, the bladder usually wakes me only once at night or only in the early morning even if I've drunk in the evening.

Why does the cranberry juice help even without bacterial evidence? Apparently, its content of powerful antioxidants strengthens the immune system. Since stress considerably weakens the body's defenses, the berry juice helps rather indirectly, quasi as a second immune system. So I got used to drinking a glass of cranberry juice in the morning, and in the evening. Or I mix a teaspoonful of powder twice a day with fruit, salad dressing or yogurt.

If we can tolerate little acidity

Some people eat too much acid with bread and cheese or sausage, without suffering directly. It is sometimes recognized that they no longer need a comb. With me it is different. If I eat only one-time bread without salad, an alkaline soup or vegetables I feel at least an hour later uncomfortable. So I can not allow myself to eat acid-producing food without buffering with green stuff or other alkaline-forming agents. For example, if I drink a glass of cranberry juice, I add some soda. It then tastes like a soda pop. Sometimes I add one tablespoon of sweet whey powder.

The most alkaline-forming fruits and vegetables are bananas, figs, papaya, fresh olives, cucumber, black radish, chestnuts, carrots, and potatoes. Legumes except for white beans are acid-forming but get a base surplus by germination. Grains, such as buckwheat, spelt, corn, and millet are neutral, all other rye varieties and rice are rich in acids.

By the way, I get a memorandum for other lapses as well: If I dare to drink too little, I feel the bladder at the latest in the evening. And if I ignore this, the kidneys tweak. If I drink two glasses of water, the pressure is gone again.

We all can learn to communicate with our body. This requires that we pay attention to its signs. Whenever the body gives a shout, we better ask: What have I done wrong?
Too much stress, too little sleep,
too much fat, too little fresh air,
did I spend too long on the computer, did I exercise too little? Over time, we can learn to recognize just what our body is missing.

Cranberry tip for bright minds

When I was writing this book in 2007, my friend Ursula Keim called me. Since she had also lived in the USA for a while, I asked her about a possible cranberry experience. She could not come up with one, but with a super-duper savings tip. I then immediately restyled my icebox and filled the undiluted cranberry juice in ice dishes. With the ice-cold red cubes, the berry juice can be portioned in an economical manner:

In the evening, place two or three cubes in a glass in the refrigerator and pour fresh water over it in the morning. These cool red berry cubes can transform each ordinary cocktail into a rattling health drink.

With an inflammation in the mouth, we can suck on it. If the eyes are reddened or aching, we push them between cotton pads and place them on the inflamed eyes. It will be best if we enjoy a bath at the same time to avoid stains. This allows us to do the same with burns and fix the red ice cotton pads, if necessary, with a bandage on the relevant places.

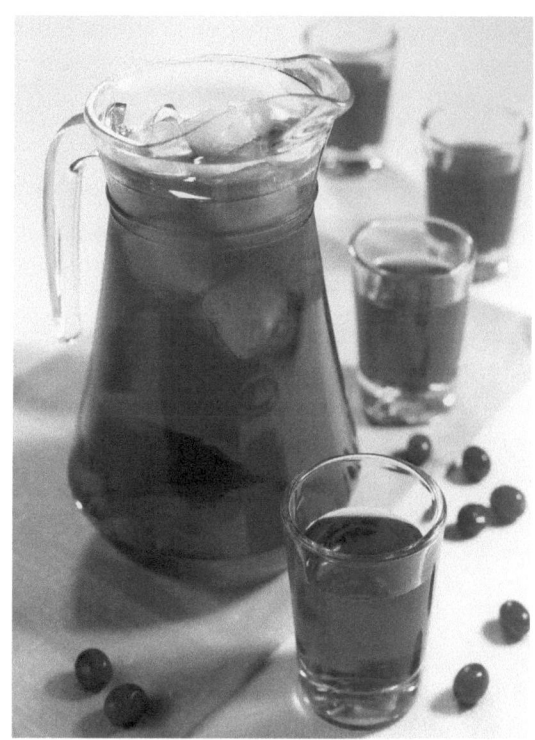

VI. REFINED RECIPES OF THE HEALTH CUISINE

The following recipes are for four people unless otherwise specified. I modified most Lucullan creations some based on original recipes of well-known cooks to support my philosophy replacing animal products with tofu, white beans or mushrooms.

If you forget to take capsules as I do, better prepare a universal mash with cranberry powder for hearty and sweet food every three to four days. The spicy variety can either be eaten raw, for example with an egg yolk as "tartar" to salads and vegetable dishes. Or you mix them with a lot of onions or fry the onions in the pan and use the mass as a base for "meat" sauces or meatballs. This saves you a lot of time, and with unexpected guests, you always have something in the fridge.

With the universal mass you can not build bombs, but knockout dishes. For the sake of simplicity mix it in a jar, with a blender.

Spicy universal mash

1 lb white beans	cooked; alternative:
½ cup chia seeds	soaked 20 min. in water mix in a blender with the following ingredients:
½ cup almond milk	
4 tbsp coconut oil	alternatively linseed oil or other organic vegetable oil
1 piece of ginger	thumb-size, peel, quarter
2 tbsp cranberry	powder
3 tbsp vegetable	seasoning, (organic or without flavor enhancer)
1 tbsp mustard	and/or
½ tsp horseradish	season with
salt and cayenne	

Tip: If the consistency is too thin, you can thicken with sesame seeds, chestnut flour or germinated sunflowers. Find out how versatile you can diversify white beans or chia seeds. If you want it as ground meat, add 2 tbsp soy and 2 tbsp tomato sauce to thicken. For a light peanut flavor, thicken the mash with soy flour and use sesame oil. With the latter two ingredients you can quickly make a tasty sauce:

1 tablespoon soy sauce on 2 tbsp sesame oil and 1 tsp cranberry powder per person. Or 1 tbsp soy sauce, 1 tbsp sesame oil and 1 tbsp cranberry sirup.

The universal mash I use fresh in the first 2 to 3 days. If on the 3rd or 4th day I still have much left, I use it with 3-4 tbsp oil and 1 cup of coconut cream in a vegetable casserole.

Sweet universal mash

½ cup chia seeds	soak 20 min. in water; mix in a blender with the following ingredients:
2 tbsp coconut	or
2 tbsp rice flour	
½ cup almond milk	
1 cup coconut whipped cream	or
2 tbsp cranberry	powder
½ organic lemon	grate the peel and add it with the juice; sweeten with ½ tsp liquid stevia

Tip: If the consistency is too thin you can add some psyllium husks or whey powder. For a peanut flavor, thicken the mash with soy flour using sesame oil.

The sweet universal mash you can use fresh in the first 2 to 3 days. If on the 3rd or 4th day you still have much left, mix it with 3-4 tbsp oil and ½ cup of coconut cream to make a cake. You can also fold in dried cranberries and small-cut fruits into a dough. Or put it in a springform pan, sprinkle soaked cranberries and 2 tbsp of almonds, put a few butter flasks on it and bake the whole thing at 300°F for about 1½ hours in the oven.

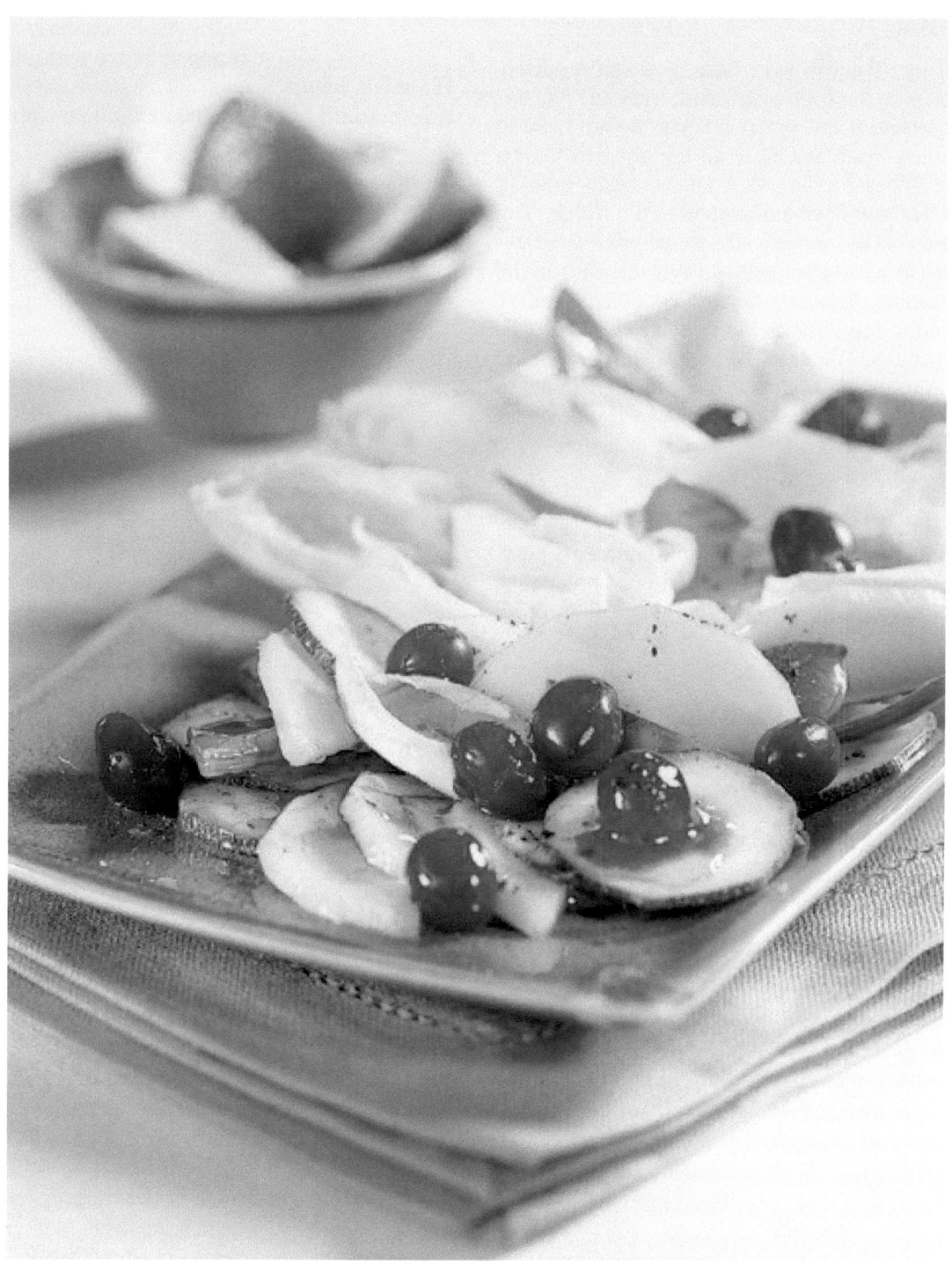

Salads

If you want to save time, you can regularly prepare the following salad dressing. The advantage of this practice is you do not have to touch, open and close all the jars and bottles of spices every time. A salad is ready quickly when you have a marinade in the fridge. You are also more motivated to eat your salad every day and to prepare a vegetable dish in the evening. You only need to cook the greenery and to season with the dressing. The ingredients can, of course, be to suit your individual taste. In addition, you can add ingredients to support your health, such as garlic for better circulation or yellow linseed to promote digestion.

Cranberry dressing

Squeeze fresh vegetable oil, cranberry powder, salt, pepper, mustard and/or horseradish powder, turmeric, organic vegetable broth powder, fresh and/or dried herbs into a screwed glass; shake.

Asparagus salad with "ham" strips

1 lb green asparagus	peel bottom third part; for 8 minutes simmer in salt water
1 head green salad	wash and let drip off; cut
4-inch baguette	in thin slices and roast
4 slices tofu	cut into wide strips; alternatively, use pickled wild salmon

For the sauce:

1 small onion	peel, cut in half, finely dice; steam with
3 tbsp cranberries in	
3 tbsp olive/canola oil	
1 tbsp sheep yogurt	or whey concentrate; let it boil down; remove from heat; chop
1 tbsp cranberries	
1 bn mixed herbs	clean, remove thick stalks; leaves coarsely chopped; puree with
125 ml of yogurt	and
1 tsp mustard	in a blender; dilute with
3-4 tbsp water	mix the herbal cream and cranberry onion mixture; season with
salt and cayenne	arrange asparagus and lettuce, spread the sauce

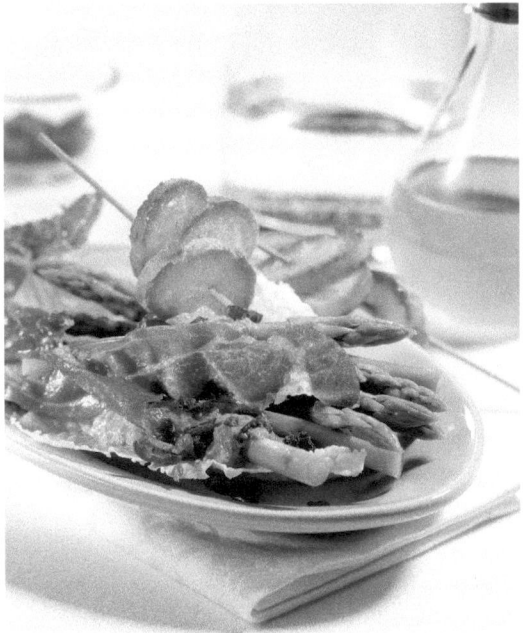

over it; garnish with tofu (salmon) and baguette slices; sprinkle chopped cranberries over the salad.

Tip: Salad sauces with yogurt or clabbered milk are fresh and aromatic and need only a little oil. No vinegar is necessary due to the natural acidity of these dairy products.

Cranberry vegetable salad

1/4 lb sugar snaps	wash in salt water blanch; let drain well
2 heads of chicory	set aside a few leaves

	halve alongside, cut finger width stripes; wash and cut in slices: peel pulp; divide elongate; slowly heat with in a pan; add 2 tbsp water and let simmer 1 minute; get the cranberries out and mix them with the mango and the prepared vegetables; mix the cranberry liquid with
2 small zucchini	
1 mango	
3 oz cranberries	
2 tbsp oil	
1-2 tbsp oil	and the juice of
2 limes	into a dressing; add coarse
pepper, salt	and some
maple sirup	stir under the salad; decorate with chicory leaves

Millet and cranberry salad

1 cup millet	wash hot in a sieve; cook gently with
3 cups water	and
½ tsp salt	for 8 min.; switch off; let swell for 15 min.
1 bn green onions	wash, finely dice, cut green parts in rings; saute in
2 tbsp olive/rapseed oil	until glassy
2 oz cranberry	dried; bring to the boil in
1 cup of water	let simmer for 5 min.
½ bn fresh mint	wash; chop; dry roast
2 oz pine nuts	fillet
2 grapefruits	catch the juice; stir
6 oz sheep yogurt,	grapefruit juice, and
2 tbsp lemon juice	until smooth; fold in green onions, fillets, and fresh mint; sweeten with
2 drops of stevia	season with
salt & cayenne	or turmeric; mix with the millet

Red, raw vegetable salad

3 cups red cabbage	either cut or grated
1 ts carrots	grated rubbed
½ cup onions	cut fine rings
½ cup cranberries	roughly chopped, retain a few
3 tbsp sunflower	seeds heat in pan for 10 minutes, stir several times; mix 2 tbsp of it with all other ingredients
3 tbsp lemon juice	and
3 tbsp mayonnaise	organic or homemade with egg yolk, stir in 3 tbsp of

oil drop-wise in a bowl, add mustard, salt, and pepper; garnish with halved cranberries and remaining sunflower seeds

Spinach salad with cranberries

10 oz spinach	wash, sort out
½ red peppers	wash; cut in very fine cubes (keep 1 tbsp)
1 garlic clove	peel and strain it through a press; with the garlic mash
4 tbsp olive oil	and
2 tbsp yogurt	preferably sheep's yogurt do a dressing; season with
salt & cayenne	in a small casserole roast
2 oz walnuts	without fat; remove
1 tbsp oil	and
5 oz cranberries	fresh/thawed; fry in hot pan for 1 min
1 tbsp cranberries	dried, finely chopped
5 oz goat's cheese	mix with residual paprika and the chopped cranberry,

fresh pepper, and spinach with lukewarm dressing, walnuts, and roasted cranberries, serve with whole wheat toast or pita

Taboulé

¼ l vegetable broth	boil; stir in
4 oz of bulgur	cover and leave it to swell for 15 minutes
1 cup cranberries	fresh or thawed, halving or quartering; mix along

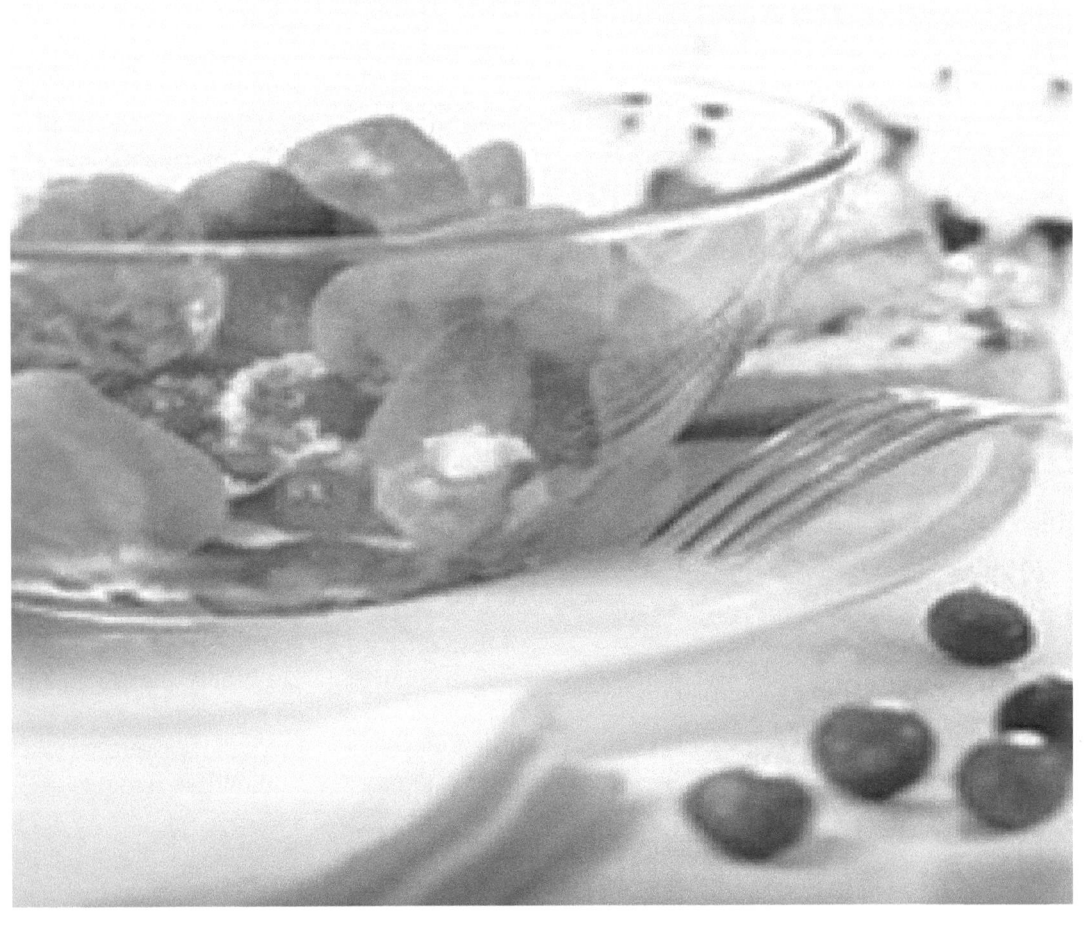

Soups, snacks, and appetizers

Ajoli-Cranioli

	with
2 green onions	cut into ½ cm thick rings
1 green pepper	cut into fine strips
1 bn parsley	remove the stalks
½ bn cilantro	remove the stalks
3 peppermint branches, remove the stalks; mix juice of	
2 lemons	and
3 tbsp olive oil	season with
salt & cayenne	serve on a bed of lettuce; trim with
10 -12 olives	

4-6 garlic cloves	cut up small, puree with
2 tbsp cranberry	jam or preserves; instead cranberry powder (2-3 cps)
5 drops stevia	
2 tbsp organic lemon juice	
1 tsp sea salt	and
1 pinch cayenne	in a blender; add very slowly
¼ cup olive oil	until the desired consistency is reached; season with
1 tsp mustard	serve with bread below

Avocado puree with

¼ tsp sea/stone salt	
1 pinch cayenne	
1 tbsp vegetable broth powder	
1 tbsp lemon juice and	
2 tbsp olive oil	to make a marinade; add the flesh of 1 avocado crushed with a fork; mix with
4 oz sheep yogurt	
4 oz cranberries	fresh or defrosted; chop roughly (leave 10 whole)

and work in; garnish with whole or halved cranberries and a sprig of mint. To this tastes the flatbread on this page.

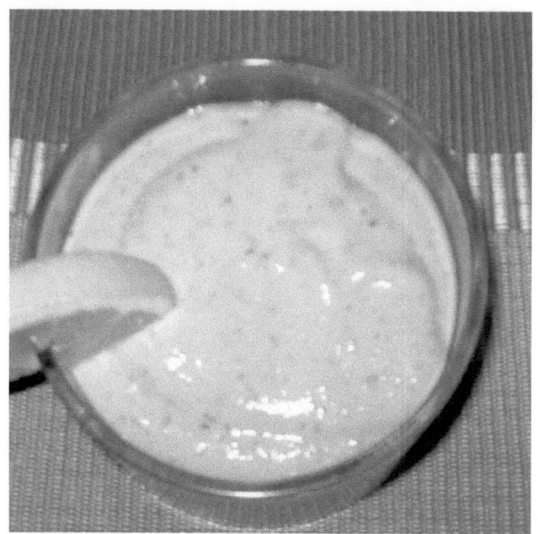

Carrot soup with cranberries and pita

3 tbsp cranberries soak 1 tbsp in 2 tbsp boiling water for 20 minutes, strain, collect the liquid; chop remaining 2 tbsp; wash and peel

2 potatoes	medium-sized and
3 oz parsley root	or add other tuber vegetables to the soup; wash, peel, dice
1 large onion	saute in
2 tbsp butter	
1 tsp of curry	and
1 tsp turmeric	also briefly saute the vegetables and chopped cranberries; pour in
750 ml broth	simmer the vegetables until soft, puree; brown the soaked cranberries slightly in the remaining butter; add liquid and allow to boil; add berries to the soup; fold in
7 oz sweet cream	heat soup again; add
1 large onion	saute in
2 tbsp butter	
1 tsp of curry	and
1 tsp turmeric	also briefly saute the vegetables and chopped cranberries; pour in
750 ml broth	simmer the vegetables until soft, puree; brown the soaked cranberries slightly in the remaining butter; add liquid and allow to boil; add berries to the soup; fold in
7 oz sweet cream	heat soup again; add
salt & cayenne	and
1 pinch licorice	powder and serve with chopped chives

Flatbread (chapati)

1 lb whole grain flour	put into a bowl, make a little hollow in the center; add
2 tbsp butter/oil	stir in little by little
6 oz warm water	knead for approx 10 min. to form a soft and elastic

dough; form into a ball; wrap it in a damp kitchen towel or wrapping film and allow to

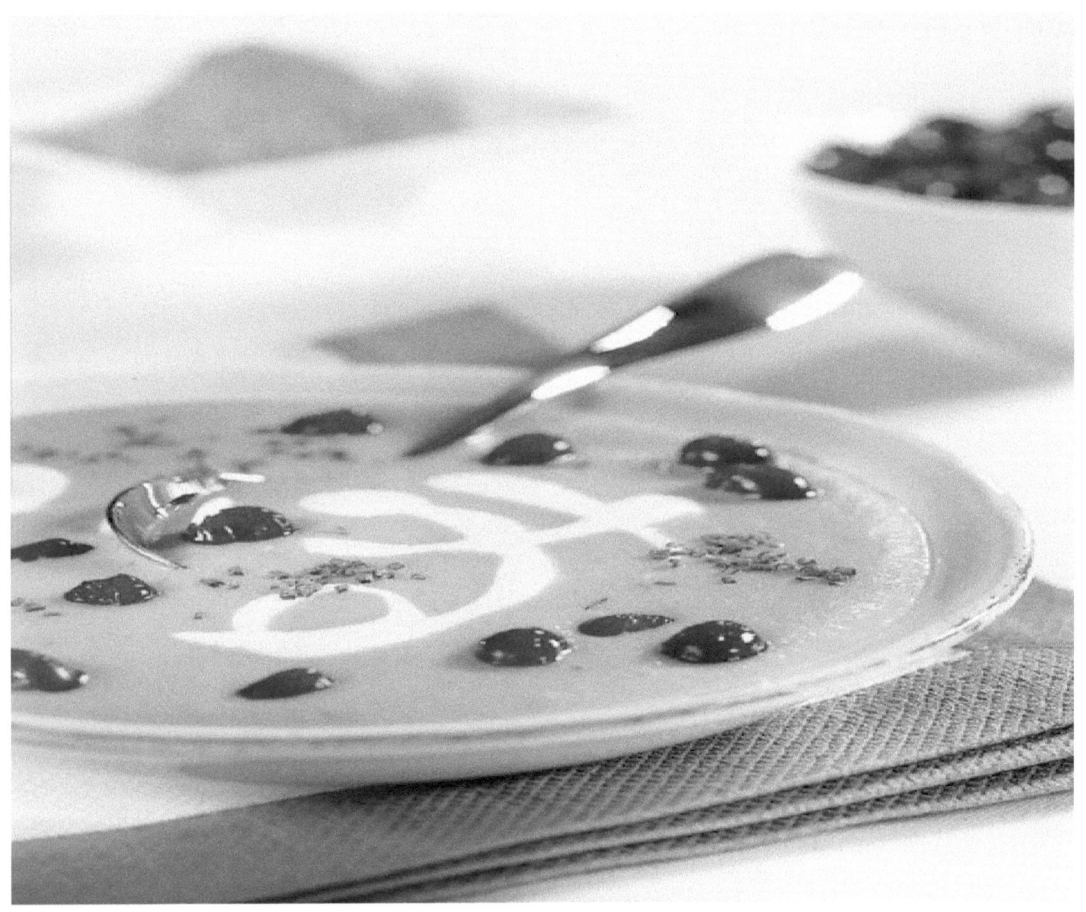

for a ½ hour minimum. Divide the dough into 12 portions, forming them into small balls; roll round and thin on a floured board. After rolling out, place next to each other; cover with a damp cloth so they do not dry out. Heat a pan for 5 minutes at medium heat; bake chapati dry until underside has white spots and top side bubbles; turn; bake until top side has brown spots; wipe out the flour from the pan between each baking step; keep the finished chapatis in a closed pot so they do not cool too quickly and dry out; best prepare them shortly before serving or freeze as a stock.

Green spelt soup

5 oz solid tofu	finely dice; mix with
½ tsp herbal salt	
cayenne & turmeric	
1 pinch mustard flour	
2 tbsp olive/rapeseed oil	and
1 tbsp liquid seasoning	refrigerate
1 cup green spelt	soak overnight in cold water; strain; simmer with
3-4 cups water	and
½ tsp salt	for 1 hour in
2 tbsp olive/rapeseed oil	
1 onion finely chopped	and
1 clove of garlic	press out; brown

for 3-4 minutes deglaze with the green spelt soup, simmer for a few minutes; in the meantime add

2 tbsp cranberries	
1 tbsp parsley	and
1 tbsp chervil	chop finely
1 tbsp of chives	cut finely; add
1 cup rice milk	with the tofu, the chopped cranberries and herbs to the soup

Kichari with cranberries

1 cup rice	basmati parboiled; wash together with
½ cup mung bean	(dal) in a sieve under flowing water; clean
1 large carrot	and
½ fennel bulb	peel and cut in small cubes
1 tbsp ghee	(clarified butter) heat in a pot; add
1 pinch cayenne	
½ tbsp cumin	
¼ tbsp turmeric	and
¼ tsp coriander	(ground); roast briefly; stir-fry vegetables; add rice and dal; pour on
3-4 cups water	heat; when the kichari begins to cook, add
1 tsp salt	simmer lightly about 10 minutes; add
½ cup cranberries	simmer another 10 min.; when the liquid has thickened add fresh basil

Roasted and salted cranberries

Pull cranberries through beaten egg whites, roll in the sesame flour and roast in a well-coated pan with little oil at a mild heat; salt lightly; serve either still warm or cooled.

Naan bread

500 g spelt flour	mix with
2 tsp baking soda	and
1 tsp salt	in a bowl; mix
1 tbsp concentrated	butter or oil; add
125 g yogurt	while stirring; add
250 g of oat milk	gradually stir in until a soft dough is produced; leave the rest in

a warm place for 2 hours with a damp cloth; divide the dough into 8 portions; roll each into an oval, brush with water; with the moist side bake in greased pan or spread with butter or oil; bake in a preheated oven at 356°F for about 10 minutes.

Sweet-and-sour cranberry coconut soup

1 thumb-sized ginger	piece peel, rub or chop finely
1-2 chili peppers	cut fine rings
4 oz shallots	peel, cut into slices
4 oz fresh cranberries	or 2 oz dried; roast in
2 tbsp sesame oil	often stir; deglaze with
400 ml coconut milk	stock up with
½ l vegetable broth	or water; bring to a boil
1 lb courgettes	wash, dice, add on; simmer for 15 min. over low heat; add
7 oz litchis fresh	peeled or from a can to the soup
½ bn cilantro	wash, dry, chop; add
6 tbsp soy sauce	to the soup squeeze out
1 lime	add and season with herbal salt

Tip: The soup tastes particularly good with roasted walnuts. Mix 3-4 oz walnut kernels with 1 teaspoon of protein, a hefty pinch of sea salt and ½ teaspoon of chopped cumin and coriander seeds. Roast in the oven at 180 degrees (circulating air 320 degrees) on a baking sheet for 10 minutes. Remove from the oven and chop roughly. Spread some of the nuts over the soup and serve the rest.

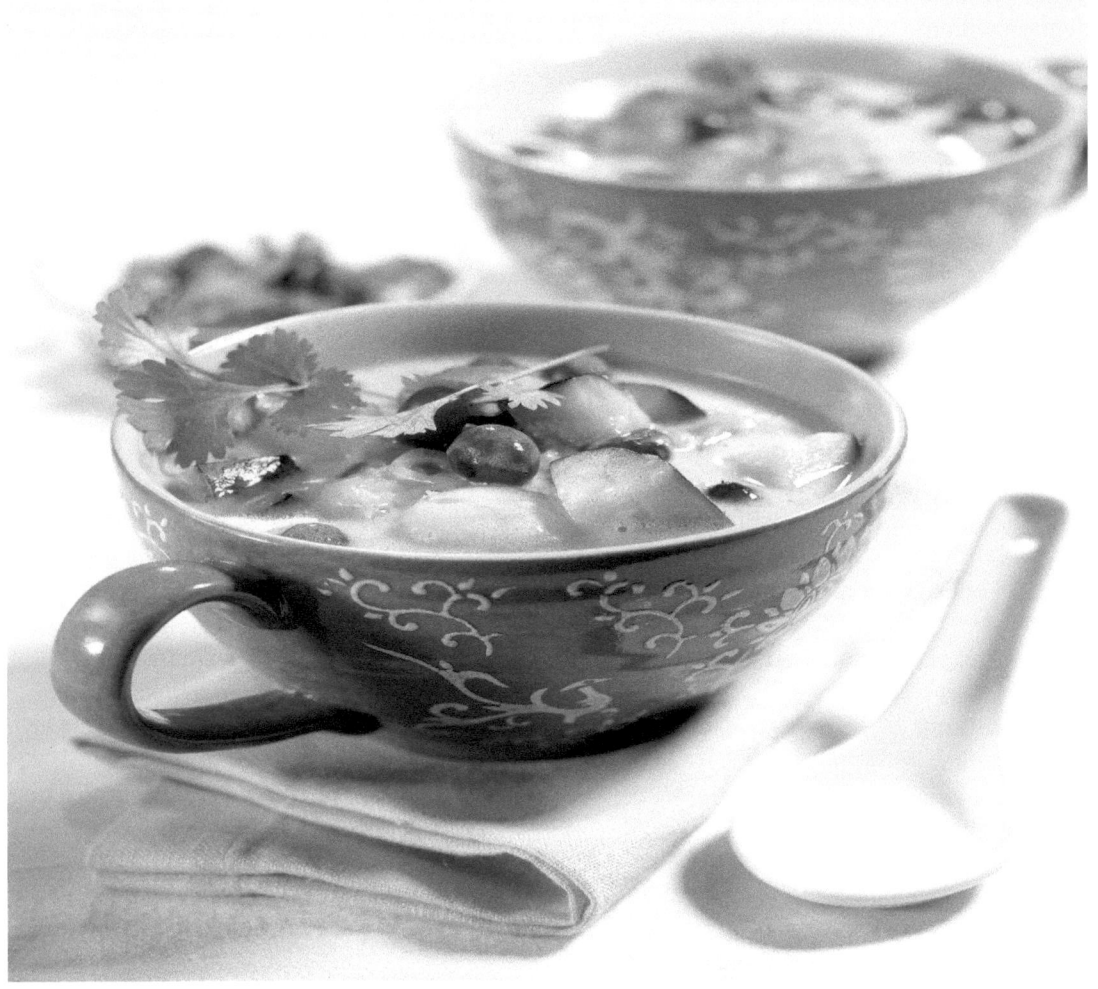

Main courts without beheading

Apple curd casserole with cranberries

Ingredients for two
1-2 sour apples   wash, peel, cut in slices; marinate
3 tbsp cranberries dried (or 1 cup fresh) with
2 tbsp orange juice mix
2 eggs
2 oz concentrated pear juice
8 oz low-fat quark
¼ organic lemon peel
1 pinch of sea salt
3 tbsp of semolina   and
1 tsp baking soda   until it attains a creamy consistency; fold in the fruits; preheat oven to 356 degrees. Grease fireproof form with 1 tsp of oil. Fill in the curd-fruit mass. Bake for about 40 minutes in the oven. It tastes great with a vanilla sauce.

Aubergine cranberry pizza

Ingredients for 2 people
1 small eggplant	wash along with
2 small courgettes	cut both into thin slices
1 tbsp tomato paste	organic brand, and
1 can tomatoes	or 2 fresh tomatoes, chop; mix with
1 tsp herbal salt	add each
1 tbsp oregano, thyme, basil & rosemary	

For the dough:
4 oz low-fat curd	whisk with
2 small eggs	
2-3 tbsp olive oil	and
½ tsp the sea salt	in a blender; mix with
1½ cup flour	
1 tsp baking soda	sift and stir in the curd-oil mixture.

If the dough is too firm, add water; work it with the kneading hooks until it comes away from the bowl; roll the dough out on a greased baking tray; spread the tomato sauce on the pastry; place the aubergine and the apple slices on top.

½ cup cranberries	fresh, defrosted or 2 tbsp dried, roughly chopped; spread over the veggies
5 oz sheep's cheese	crumble over it; in the pre-heated oven bake

pizza for 30 minutes at 338°F

Tip: If the curd dough is not crispy enough, you can also use the sourdough described under cranberry nut bread.

Cranberry fresh cheese balls on salad

2 oz cranberries	chop
2 tbsp mixed herbs	chop; mix with
2 tbsp sesame seeds	in a soup bowl
7 oz soft goat cheese	season with
sea salt & cayenne	with a spoon cut nut-sized portions; sluff

them off an turn them in the soup bowl with the cranberry sesame mixture; form into balls; keep them in the refrigerator until they are served

3 oz lamb's lettuce	alternatively 1 small head of frisée lettuce; wash
1 grapefruit peel	filet, remove the white skin (alternate with 2 oranges or ½ pineapple)

For the sauce:
4 tbsp cranberry juice	mix with
4 tbsp sour cream	
1 tsp grated horseradish	and
1-2 tbsp nut/sesame oil	season with
salt and pepper;	put the salad, fruit and cheese balls on

4 plates; sprinkle the sauce over the lettuce leaves

Tip: The fresh cheese balls can also be placed in small praline cups decorating cold buffets.

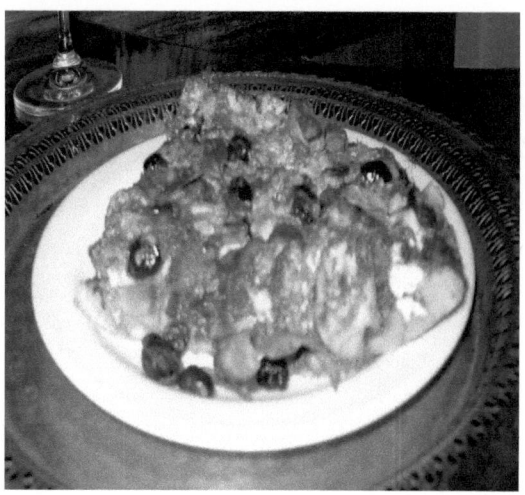

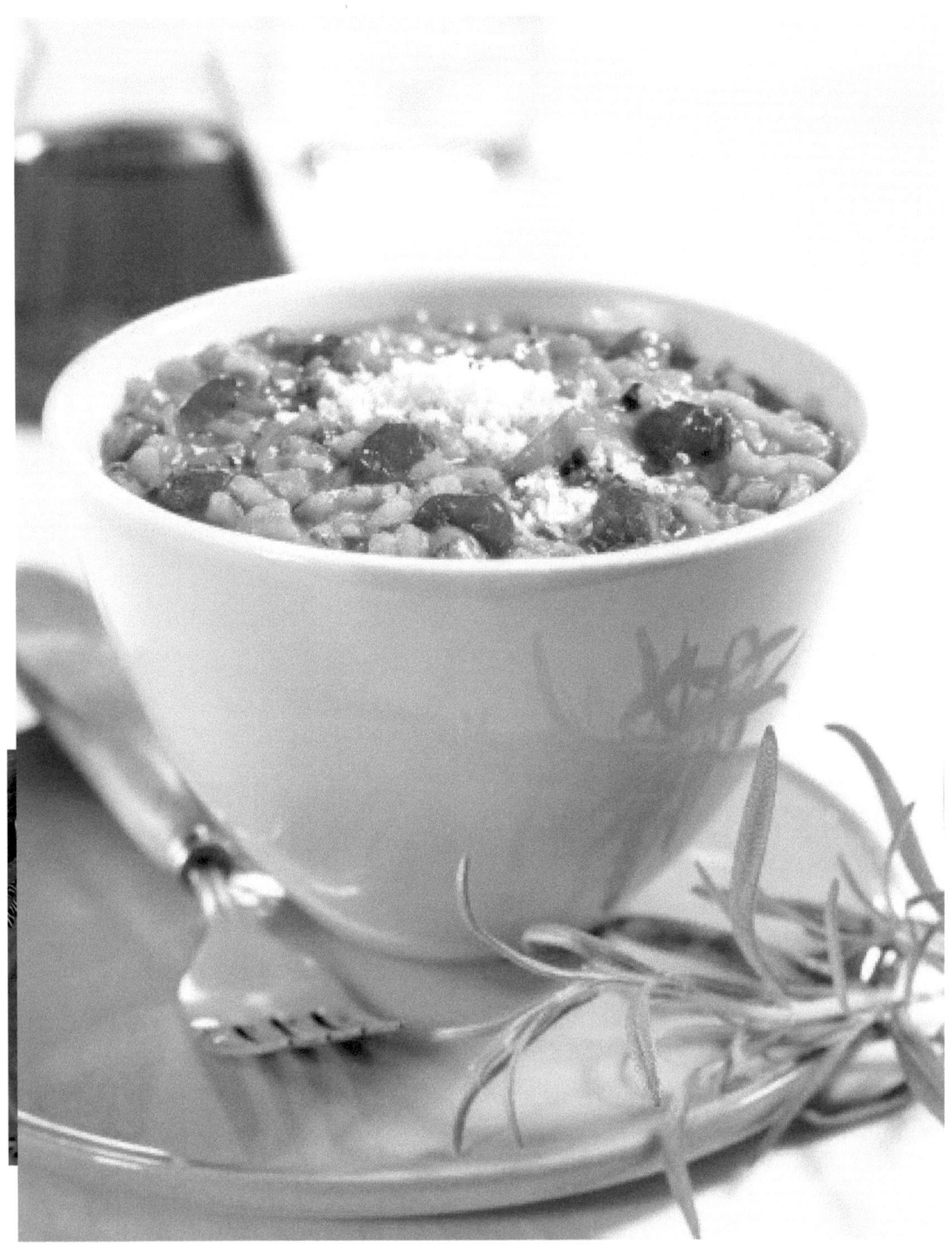

Cranberry nut bread

1 lb rye flour	mix with
1½ cup water	warm
30 g sourdough	and
1 level tsp salt	and stir 5 min with the kneading hook to a firm smooth dough; fold in
3 oz cranberries	(roughly chopped) and
3 oz hazel/walnuts	sprinkle thickly with flour; allow the dough to rise; shape bread, place in-

to the baking tin; allow to rise again; spread some lukewarm water on; bake in a preheated oven at 338°F until no more dough sticks to a rod or needle inserted into the center

Cannelloni rolls

For the dough:

2 cups flour	sieve on the worktop; make a depression in the center; add
3 eggs	
2 tbsp olive oil and	
¾ tsp sea salt	and mix with a fork; progressively mix in flour; by

hand, add more flour and knead the dough for about 15 minutes or use the faster electric kneading hook, but the last minute it's better to knead by hand. If the dough is too dry add some water or olive oil; wrap the dough ball in cling film and place in the refrigerator for 1 hour, then thinly roll out the dough and cut 4 x 4 inch large layers

For the filling:

1 lb white beans	together with
3 tbsp mixed herbs	
1 tsp salt	and
2 tbsp liquid seasoning	(organic) let stand for a short while, then puree
¼ cup cranberries	fresh or frozen roughly chopped
5 tbsp fresh cheese	
5 tbsp ground almonds	press
3-4 garlic cloves	mix together with
1 tbsp herbs of Provence	
40 g of Parmesan	and
salt and pepper	spread the mixture on the dough layers; roll

it up; grease a casserole dish, place the dough rolls next to each other

For the sauce:

1 large onion	dice
2 tbsp coconut oil	fry in
2 lb tomatoes	put in boiling water, skin add to the onions; add
1 tbsp vegetable broth powder and	
1 tsp basil (dried)	season with
herbal salt & cayenne	let simmer some min.

pour over the cannelloni and bake at 356°F for about 30 minutes; jf necessary add sauce

Cranberry pumpkin risotto

1 lb Hokkaido pumpkin	remove seeds; dice
1 onion	and
2-3 cloves garlic	finely diced; wash
1 sprig rosemary	remove needles and chop; bring
2½ cups cranberry juice	and
1¾ cups vegetable broth	in a saucepan to a boil; switch back to the lowest heat; heat
2-3 tbsp olive oil	in a large pot; steam
5 oz cranberries	with the prepared ingredients; flavor with
sea salt & cayenne	add
8 oz of risotto rice	sauté briefly together; stew one-third of the

juice-broth mixture into the pot. Cook risotto over medium heat for 20 minutes; stir occasionally; gradually add the remaining broth. The risotto should be creamy, but the rice still firm to the bite; stir

4 tbsp chopped parsley	
4 tbsp fresh Parmesan	and
1-2 tbsp butter I	into the risotto, season

to taste and serve immediately. Serve with a green salad and with walnuts.

Tip: The tasty pumpkin resembles the shape of a fresh fig. It contains more carotenoids than carrots and is particularly easy to process: the vigorous orange-colored skin of the Hokkaido pumpkin does not need to be removed. It is soft when cooked and can be eaten. A hollow sound when tapping on it shows it is ripe. It can be stored at a temperature of 54 to 62°F in a dry and well-ventilated room for up to one year.

Fried pumpkin with dried cranberries

Ingredients for two

½ cup cranberries	simmer in
4 oz orange juice	at low heat for 10 min.
2/3 lb pumpkin	cut the meat into slices
1 sour apple	peel dice, mix with the cranberries and
thyme leaves	(2 stems); peel
1 onion	dice and sauté in
2 tbsp coconut oil	add cranberry mixture; steam 3 min; season with
ginger or turmeric	season with
salt and cayenne	let cool down; roast pumpkin meat in the remaining oil roast meat; deglaze with
50 ml of the broth	and the remaining juice; simmer for 10 min.; season with
salt & cayenne	arrange the pumpkin with the cranberry sauce

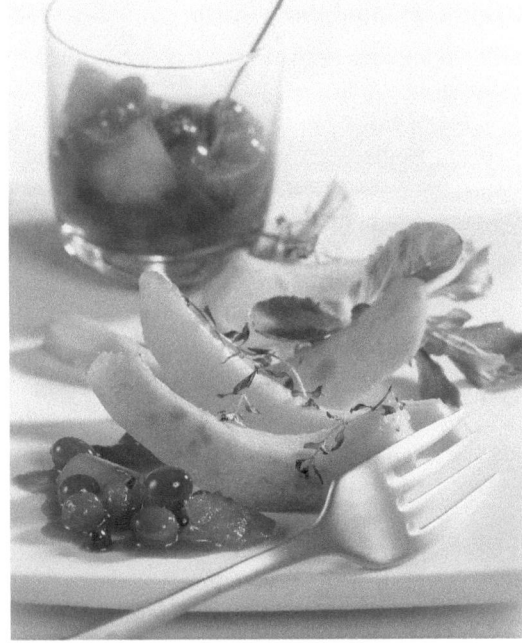

"Meat" loaf

1 lb tofu	mash
1 large onion	chop finely
1-2 eggs	
1-2 tsp mustard	soak
2 slices toast	(whole grain) in
5 tbsp rice milk	mix with all above ingredients; add
1 tbsp parsley	
1 tbsp thyme	
1 tsp herbal salt	and
1 pinch cayenne	shape into a loaf; fill in
3 tbsp cranberries	(dried) and bake in preheated oven for 30 min.

at 320°F; serve with vegetable or salad.

Potato salad with cranberry, celery and walnuts

1½ lb potatoes	cook with little salt water for 20 min. on low heat; peel and cut them into slices; finely chop
3 oz walnuts	and roast them in a frying pan without fat
½ tin tangerines	let drip off; wash
4 celery stalks	trim; slice into fine strips
1 head frisée salad	wash; spin-dry; mix
5 oz yogurt	with
2 tbsp mayonnaise	and grated rind of
1 lime	and the juice; add

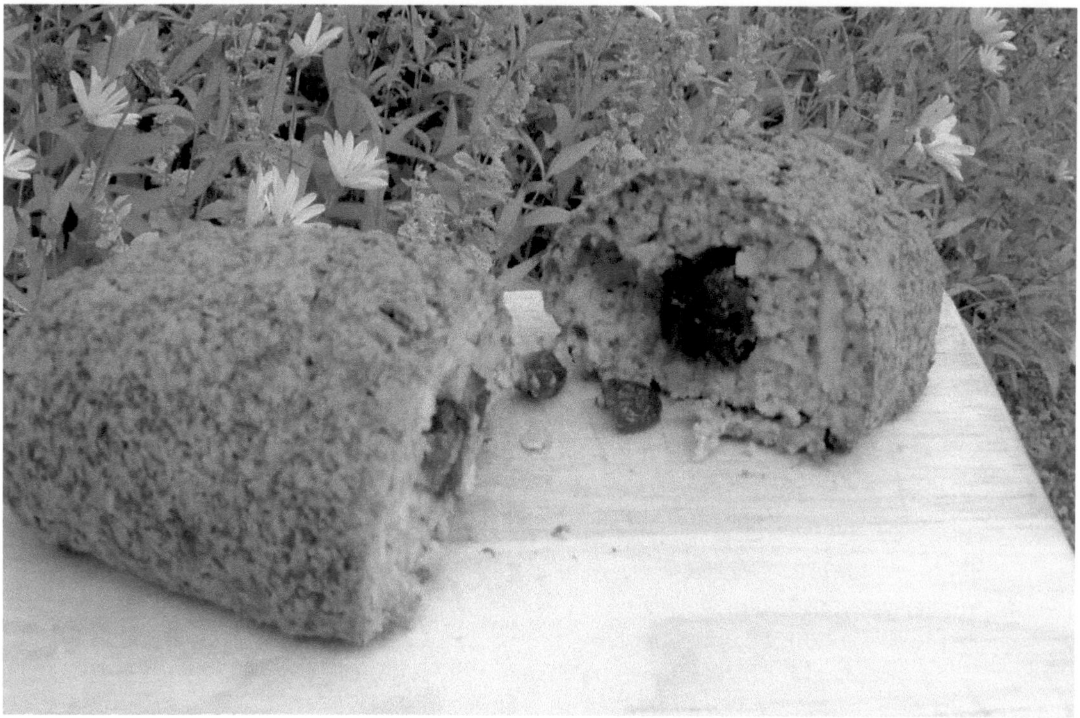

salt and cayenne	and mix with potatoes and the remaining ingredients with
2 oz cranberries	sprinkle salad with roasted walnuts

Pasta with dried cranberries

½ cup cranberries	with little water simmer for 10 minutes; cook
1 lb noodles	salt water firm to bite; drain the noodles
2 shallots	peel and finely chop
3-4 z celery stems	wash, clean and slice
3 oz walnuts	chop roughly
7 oz mackerel fillet	smoked, tear into bite-size pieces
1 bn parsley	wash, chop leaves coarsely; heat
2 tbsp coconut oil	sweat but do not brown the shallot cubes; add

	cranberries and liquid and steam until all the water has evaporated; add the celery and nuts and stew for a few minutes; add
½ cup cream	and simmer for 1 minute season with

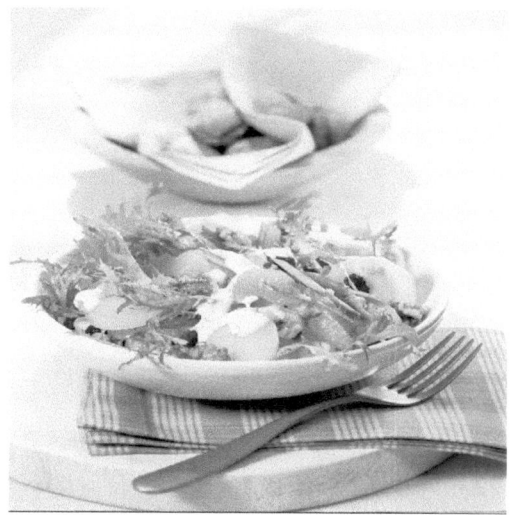

fresh pepper
1 tbsp lemon juice   and
2 drops Stevia   mix pasta with the sauce, sprinkle with the remaining parsley and serve immediately

Pizza with dried cranberries

For the dough:
1 cup flour   whole-grain, mix with
2 tbsp sourdough   starter add
1 cup water   lukewarm
2 tbsp olive oil   and
1 tsp sea salt   knead to a smooth non-sticky dough; let it rise in a warm place for about 1 hour

For the topping: bring
1/3 cup cranberries with ½ cup water to a boil; cook at low heat for 30 minutes; drain well in a sieve
2 garlic cloves   peel; finely chop; in
1 tbsp olive oil   steam until golden
1 tsp oregano and
1 tsp thyme   soak in water until

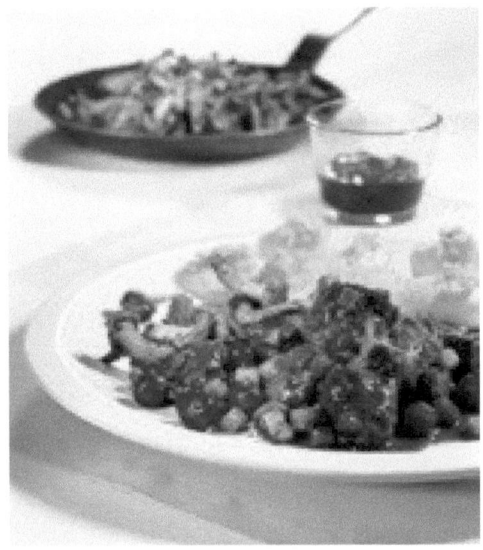

soft; add and also briefly sauté it; add
1 cup of tomato pieces (can) and the cranberries; cook for 5 minutes stirring frequently
3 tbsp tomato paste stir in; season with
sea salt & cayenne
1 onion   peel; cut into rings
5 oz vegan sausage   cut into strips
3,5 oz cheddar cheese grated
1 ball mozzarella   finely dice; mix with the cheddar cheese;

preheat oven to 420°F; lay out the sheet of baking paper; use the dough to form a thin, round cake, leaving the edge slightly thicker. Spread the cranberry mixture on the dough, cover with the sausage and onion rings. Spread the cheese on top and bake in a hot oven (lowest shelf) for about 25 minutes

½ bunch basil wash, remove the leaves from the stalk; sprinkle on the pizza

„Reh"ragout with dried cranberries and mushrooms

3-4 oz cranberries (dried); simmer in ca.
7 oz water   for 15 min.; let them drain well in a colander
4 oz soy cubes   (dried); soak in
¼ cup liquid seasoning and 1 cup of water
1 tsp juniper berries and
1 tsp fennel seeds coarsely chop or pound in a mortar; mix with
1 tbsp oil
5 shallots
4 cloves garlic   and
7 oz carrots   peel and dice; roast the "meat" in
2 tbsp coconut oil for 2-3 minutes; add
1 tbsp butter   and froth up; add liquid seasoning and
cranberries. Season with sea salt & cayenne
brown; add gradually

8-9 oz dark beer	pour on the ragout
1 cup cranberry	sirup and
1 cup of water	cook for 30 min.; in the meantime roast
8 oz boletus	or chanterelles with
1 tbsp butter	in a frying pan for 3 min. stirring frequently
1 bn chives	wash; cut in fine rolls; spread on the ragout; add
1 tbsp butter	serve with mushrooms

Spaghetti „bolognese"

4 oz g tofu granules	place in a bowl; boil water; in it skin
4 tomatoes	alternatively 1 can pizza tomatoes) and
16 oz tomatoes	strained; pour over the tofu; marinate with
½ cup cranberry sirup	
3 tbsp tomato paste	
1 tsp oregano	
salt & cayenne	and
5 tbsp liquid seasoning	pour
1 lb spaghetti	in boiling salt water
2 large onions	peel and dice
2 carrots and	
1 celery stem	remove skin; cut in thin slices or mince it in the meat grinder
2-3 tbsp olive oil	fry with the onions
3 garlic cloves	peel; finely dice and add to the vegetables; after

cooking add the tofu mash, briefly boil it up once again, turn off the heat; if the spaghetti is firm to the bite, drain the water; add some olive oil to the pot, stir; place spaghetti in deep plates and spread the sauce over it

½ bn parsley	pluck the leaves and sprinkle over each plate

Spicy reddish muffins

1 cup corn flour	mix with
1 cup of spelt flour	whole grain
¼ cup brown sugar	alternatively
5-6 drops of stevia	
2 tsp baking soda	
½ tsp herbal salt	and
¼ tbsp cayenne	in a large bowl
1 cup buttermilk	
2 tbsp butter	melted; add
2 eggs	whisked into the bowl; add
¼ cup cranberry	dried
½ cup parmesan	grated; stir in; add more buttermilk; the dough

should be easily poured into the muffin cups; bake in a pre-heated oven for 15-20 minutes, serve warm in a green salad bed.

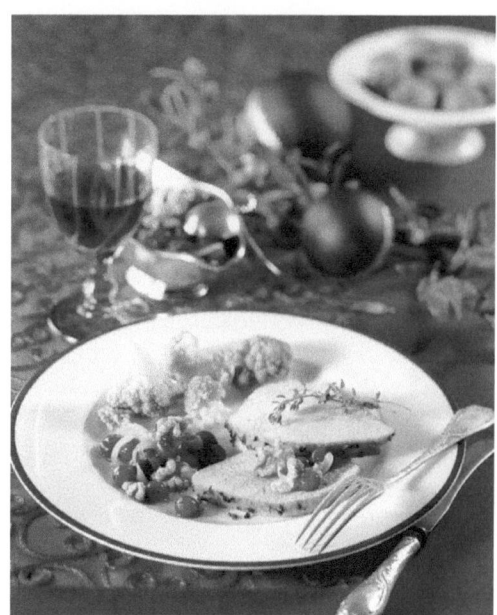

"Turkey breast" with cranberry walnut chutney

1 lb white beans	mix with
2 eggs	or
2 tbsp chia seeds	20 min. soaked in 6 tbsp

	water
1-2 tbsp oatmeal	and
1 tsp sea salt	and shape a turkey breast
1 tbsp coriander	seeds
3 cloves	
½ tsp Peppercorns	
1 slice vanilla pod	scrape out the pith and add
1 bn thyme	except for a few sprigs for the garnish, remove the leaves from the stems; put them in a mortar; crush everything;
add 2 tbsp oil	peu à peu; rub it into the "turkey breast"; marinate for 1-2 hours

For the chutney: bring
4 oz cranberries   dried, with
5 oz cranberry juice   at low heat to a boil
2 large onions   coarsely dice; steam in
1 tbsp oil   for 5 minutes; cook the cranberries with juice
1 tsp turmeric   and the juice of
½ organic lemon   6-8 minutes, stirring frequently; sprinkle
1 tsp apple pectin   over it; season with
sea salt & cayenne
3-4 oz walnuts   chop roughly, roast in a frying pan without oil; stir in; let cool; fry "turkey breast" in a dry heated oven thoroughly from all sides; pour in 1 glass of chicken fondant, add vanilla pod and let simmer with lid on for 40-45 minutes at moderate heat; remove "turkey breast"; mix
3 tbsp corn starch   with
3 tbsp vermouth   (dry), stir in the stock and boil; season with
salt & cayenne   cut turkey breast; arange together with the chutney; garnish with thyme; serve the roast sauce extra, Romanesco broccoli with walnuts and mashed potatoes.

Tip: Cloves can irritate the mucous membranes. So do not use too much of it. According to Hildegard von Bingen, they help with edema and headaches.

Zucchini boats, loaded with tofu

8 oz firm tofu	crumble with fork,
3,5 oz fresh cranberries	or 3 tbsp dried ones; chop, with
2 tbsp liquid seasoning	
150 ml tomatoes	(sieved)

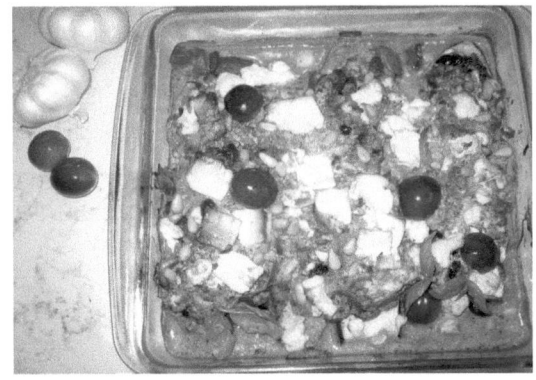

sea salt & cayenne	and
3 tbsp mixed herbs	such as oregano, thyme, basil
2 small red onions	peel and cut into quarters; cut finely, sauté 5 minutes with
½ tsp sea salt	
2 clove garlic cloves	finely dice; add to the onions; sauté another 3-4 min.; roast
1 tbsp pine nuts	without fat a few minutes stirring frequently
2 zucchini	cut in half lengthwise, hollow out; place in a fireproof form; cut the flesh into cubes; fill the zucchini boats with the tofu and the

onion-garlic mixture; stir
1 cup rice milk with
3 tsp tomato paste and mix
¼ tsp sea salt and pour over the stuffed zucchini; bake in pre-heated oven at 160 degrees for a ½ hour; sprinkle fresh basil and pine nuts over it; garnish with whole cranberries

Zucchini pancake with apple sauce

3 large potatoes finely grate
2 small zucchini roughly grate
1 large onion finely grate
3 tbsp spelt flakes or oatmeal; add
2 tbsp spelt flour and mix with
1 organic egg
8 fresh cranberries roughly chop; or use 1 tbsp dried berries: mix
1 tsp herbal salt
¼ tsp cayenne
1 dash mustard flour
1 dash nutmeg and
3 tbsp mixed herbs heat
1 tbsp olive oil in a large pan, fill in each 3 ladles full of dough, press flat, brown from both sides; clean the pan, reheat; add 1 tbsp of oil, bake the remaining fritters; serve with applesauce

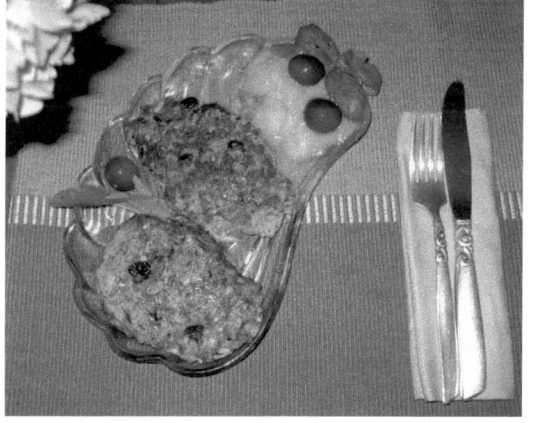

The nutmeg helps digestion. It stimulates the formation and distribution of the digestive juices, especially the bile. It also helps against ill-feelings because their ingredients Myristicin and Elemicin provide for a good mood. But beware of excessive doses!

My husband who had recently gone into the light had many times enjoyed a meal without first knowing that he could have had a pure conscience. Ever since he had seen the crowded pig transporters on our journeys to southern Europe and Morocco, he appeased his hunger for the gill breathers. If he had to catch the fish himself, that would not be an alternative either. We had never been able to choose a live chicken in Morocco and let it be slaughtered. Hubby had said, "Then I prefer only noodles with olive oil."

It is far from me to impose my philosophy on you here. However, I would like to inform you about the current agricultural policy in the name of all defenseless creatures. Here is an excerpt from my book "Migrant Birds on Wheels":

The morning hour is less profitable than the early bird proverb and the freebie highway around Valencia promise: We overtake four pigs transporting making us feel distinctly ill at ease. The animals are crowded. They can hardly move. Shocked, Peter shouts, throw away my sausages. I say, just don't buy any more. The pigs are driven through all of Europe to Morocco because the slaughtering is cheaper there. What a stress: torn from their habitual environment, crowded with strange animals. If an animal falls, it is hurt or killed by kicks of others. Schopenhauer says: "The world is not a work of art, and the animals are not a product for our use. Not mercy, but righteousness is owed to the animals."

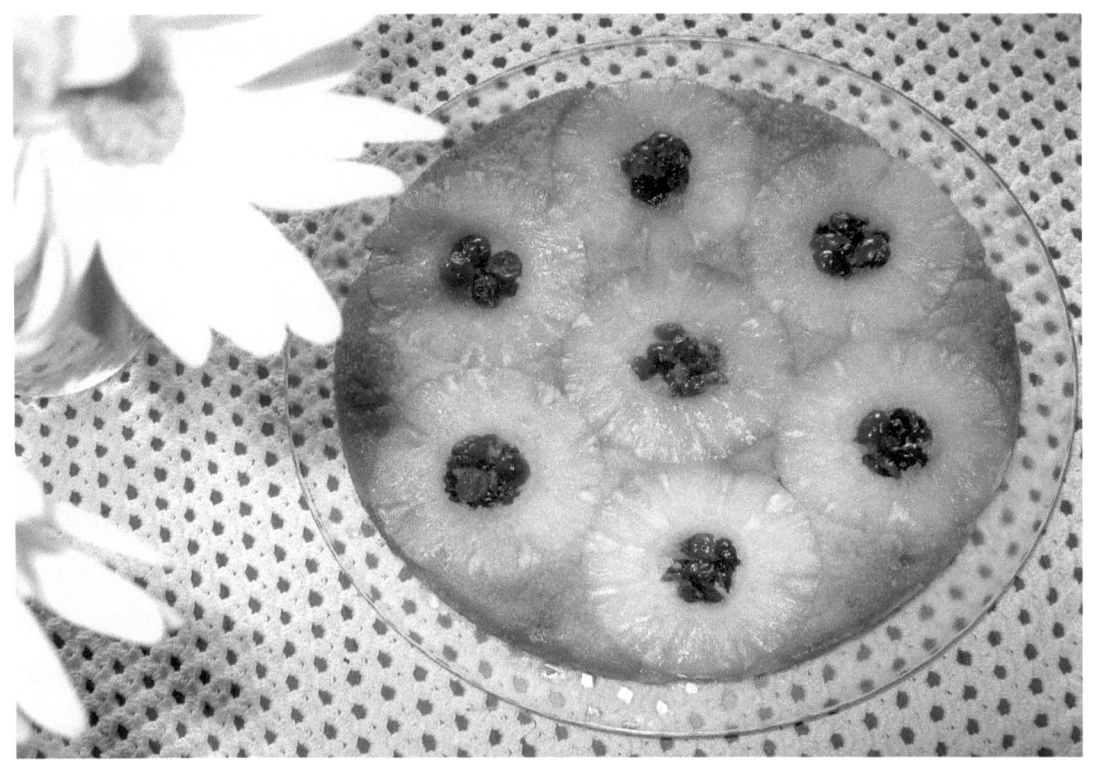

Cakes, desserts, and sweets

Instead of sugar, I use stevia or licorice powder. I also use apple pectin for fillings, drinks and as gelling aid. It's good for the heart and digestive and prevents certain cancers. Anyone who cooks with sugar, honey, agave sirup or guar gum can omit the apple pectin. The mixtures must then be boiled until they start to thicken by itself.

Ananas (pineapple) pie on the head

2 oz of cranberry	dried; soak 5 min. in litle water; melt
2 tbsp butter	in a big springorm pan at moderate heat; spread
3 tbsp brown sugar	mixed with the butter evenly over the base; lay *out*
7 pineapple slices	see photo; fill the holes with berries; whisk until frothy; melt and with
4 eggs in a bowl	
2 tbsp butter	
4-5 tbsp sugar	or 3 tbsp maple sirup until smooth; mix with; stir in
6 tbsp spelt flour	
1 tsp baking powder	

Spread the pastry over the pineapple slices. Bake cake at 320°F ½ hour or until it has a golden color; place a round cake plate on top of the pancake, throw the cake and wait a few minutes to open the mold.

Tip: If you use sweetened pineapples from the can, take a tablespoon less sugar or less of the alternative sweetener. Or use fresh or frozen cranberries, which with their tart flavor attenuate the sweetness.

Cranberry apple strudel with walnuts

For the strudel dough:
7 oz spelt flour
2 tbsp sunflower oil and mix
1 egg yolk with ½ cup lukewarm water in a bowl; on the work surface knead well for 5 minutes, then form into a ball. To prevent the dough from tearing, the ball must be ground: place hands over the dough ball and evenly circle until the dough has a velvety, smooth surface. Brush lightly with oil, cover with foil and let the dough rest in warm place for at least 30 minutes before stretching it. Alternatively: Use strudel dough from the cooling rack.

For the filling:
12 oz cranberries
7 oz sugar
2 tbsp lemon juice and
Mix 1 teaspoon of cinnamon
28 oz peeled apples, quarters, cut into slices; mix with berries; dissolve
3½ oz butter in a small pot; heat oven to 392°F (convection 356°F); grind or
3½ oz walnuts crush in mortar or grind

Put the cloth on the kitchen table, dust with flour. Roll out or stretch the dough thinly on all sides: go with both floured back of the hands under the dough and carefully pull towards the edge of the table to all sides, until the dough is very thin; cut thick dough edges. Sprinkle on the butter and the ground nuts. Spread the filling along one-third of the dough. To roll up, lift the cloth and roll the strudel towards the free dough side; with the seam down on a greased baking tray, spread with butter and bake for 30 minutes golden brown; butter two or three times; sprinkle with icing sugar and serve with whipped cream.

Cranberry almond bar

1 cup cranberries (dried) soak in
4 tbsp cranberry sirup with
1 cup raisins
½ cup almonds (ground)
3 tbsp whey powder and
1 tbsp cranberry powder in a blender; sweeten with stevia, if desired; spread onto a baking parchment lined baking sheet; dry at 122°F in the oven (keep the oven door open with a cooking spoon) or let it dry in the summer sun; cut into any desired pieces

Cranberry chocolate delight

For 1-2 persons:
3 tbsp organic butter alternatively coconut cream; bring along with
2 tbsp cocoa powder to a brief boil; remove from heat
1 oz cranberries (dried) and to sweeten
½ tsp stevia spread on the bottom of a square cake form; put in the refrigerator. If you don't want to wait, you can enjoy the mash immediately as a mousse au chocolate with 1-2 tbsp whipping cream. If you are not afraid of the bird flu, you can also refine it with a fresh organic egg yolk. With egg liqueur, you are on the safe side, at least as far as the avian influenza is concerned.

Cranberry jelly place

24 oz cranberries in a saucepan; cover them with water and cook for 15 minutes until tender; add
14-16 oz sugar and let it simmer until the liquid turns to a thick syrup. From time to time test for a set. Place the jam in clean screw top jars; close them and let them cool head down.

Cranberry sauce

2 cups cranberries (fresh or frozen) boil with in a saucepan; add
½ cup water
4 tbsp red wine (dry); simmer 10 min. or until the berries burst; slowly stir in
1 tsp apple pectin (health food store); sweeten with
½ - 1 tsp stevia

The sauce can be used immediately or stored in a refrigerator for up to two weeks.

Cranberry sorbet

1 organic orange   rinse under hot water; grate half of the peel and press out the juice
10 oz cranberry juice and
5 oz of cranberries (fresh or frozen) bring to a boil while stirring; stir in the orange juice and the grated peel; spread
1 tsp apple pectin   over it with stirring; let cool; sweeten with
½ - 1tsp stevia   finely puree the mixture, put in a cold-proof dish and place in the freezer compartment. After about an hour, thoroughly stir the mixture well and place in the freezer compartment. Repeat the procedure 2-3 times. Fill the sorbet 15 min. before serving in well-chilled glasses

Cranberry walnut muffin

<u>Ingredients for about 16 pieces:</u>
5 oz spelt whole grain flour mix with
1 tsp baking powder and
½ tsp salt   and pass thru a sieve; beat
3 eggs   fold with
5 oz sheep yogurt   and
6 oz maple sirup   gradually into the flour mix; fold in
2 oz chopped walnuts and
3 oz cranberries   oil a muffin tin with
1 tbsp canola oil   fill two-thirds with the dough; bake
at 392°F top/bottom heat (356° F circulating air) for about 25 to 30 minutes

Fruity soft ice cream

3 oz of cranberry sirup mix with
¼ tsp stevia   and freeze in a sandwich bag, eat it as it is or puree with
2 tbsp vanilla ice cream

Fruit ice cream with nut

5 oz raspberries   fresh or frozen; keep some for garnishing
3 ½ oz cranberries   fresh or frozen, keep 3 for garnishing and place in a freezer bag overnight in the freezer; then puree together with
½ cup sweet cream   or coconut cream for a few minutes; crush
2 tbsp walnuts   in the mortar; or fold chopped hazelnuts, pistachios, pine nuts or coconut chips into the mash; sweeten with stevia

Papaya pep up   (probiotic)
¼ papaya   and
2 oz cranberries   fresh or frozen, mix with
1 ½ cup rice milk   in the mixer
½ tsp FOS   or 1 capsule (fructooligosaccharides can stimulate your bifidobacteria in the colon; sweeten with
2-3 drops stevia

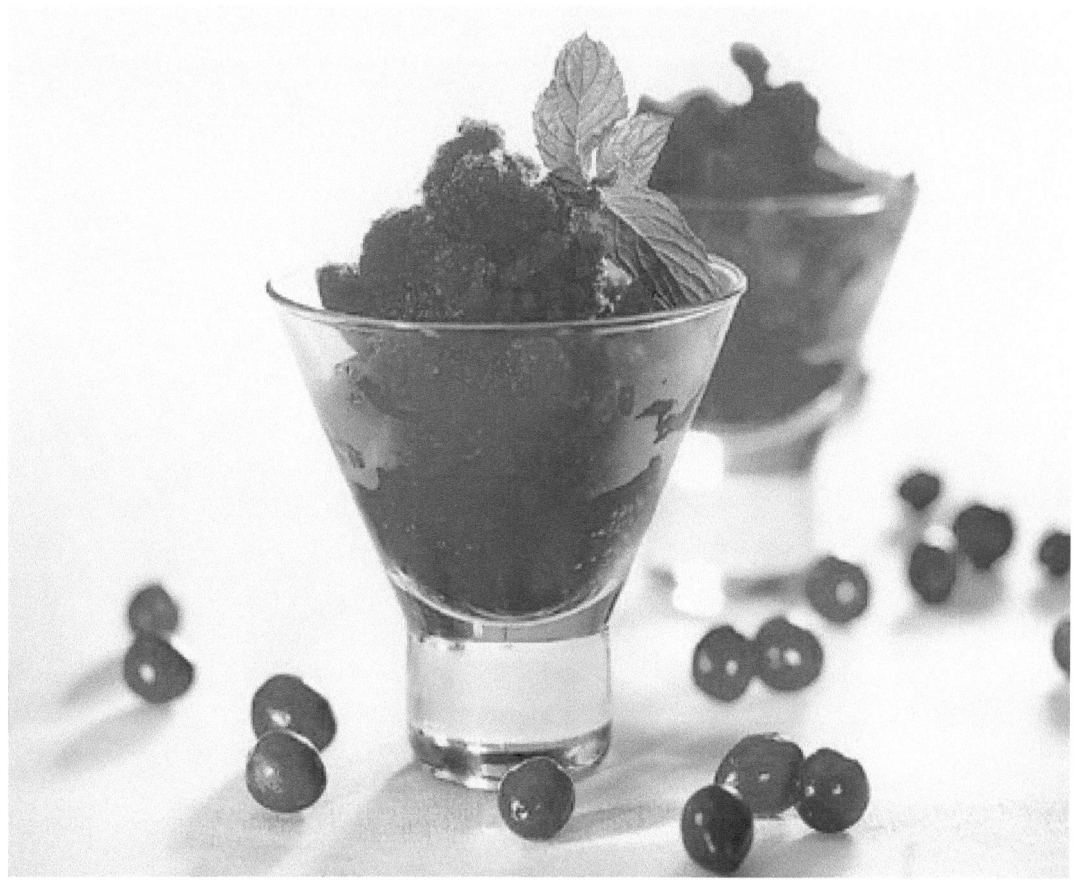

Chocolate cranberry nut cake

7 oz sweet butter	melt in a pot over low heat; add
3 tbsp cocoa	boil up briefly; allow cooling; whisk
4 eggs	or beat egg whites extra
2 tsp vanilla sugar	mix with
1 tsp baking soda	and
1½ cup spelt flour	crush
1½ cups nuts	(walnuts or pecans) in the mortar; keep some

whole nuts and add the rest to the dough; mix the chocolate-butter mixture with the dough; fill in a buttered box shaped cake form; decorate with walnuts; bake at 160° C for 1 hour and 20 minutes in a preheated oven

Tip: The cake is twice as high when you beat the egg whites separately and fold it in the dough. You can also cut it one or two times and make a cranberry cream filling: Beat 200 ml whipping cream, add 1 tsp apple pectin; fill in half the mixture, pour the other half over the cake; sprinkle coarsely chopped cranberries on top.

Beat 200 ml whipping cream, add 1 tsp apple pectin; fill in half the mixture, pour the other half over the cake; sprinkle coarsely chopped cranberries on top.

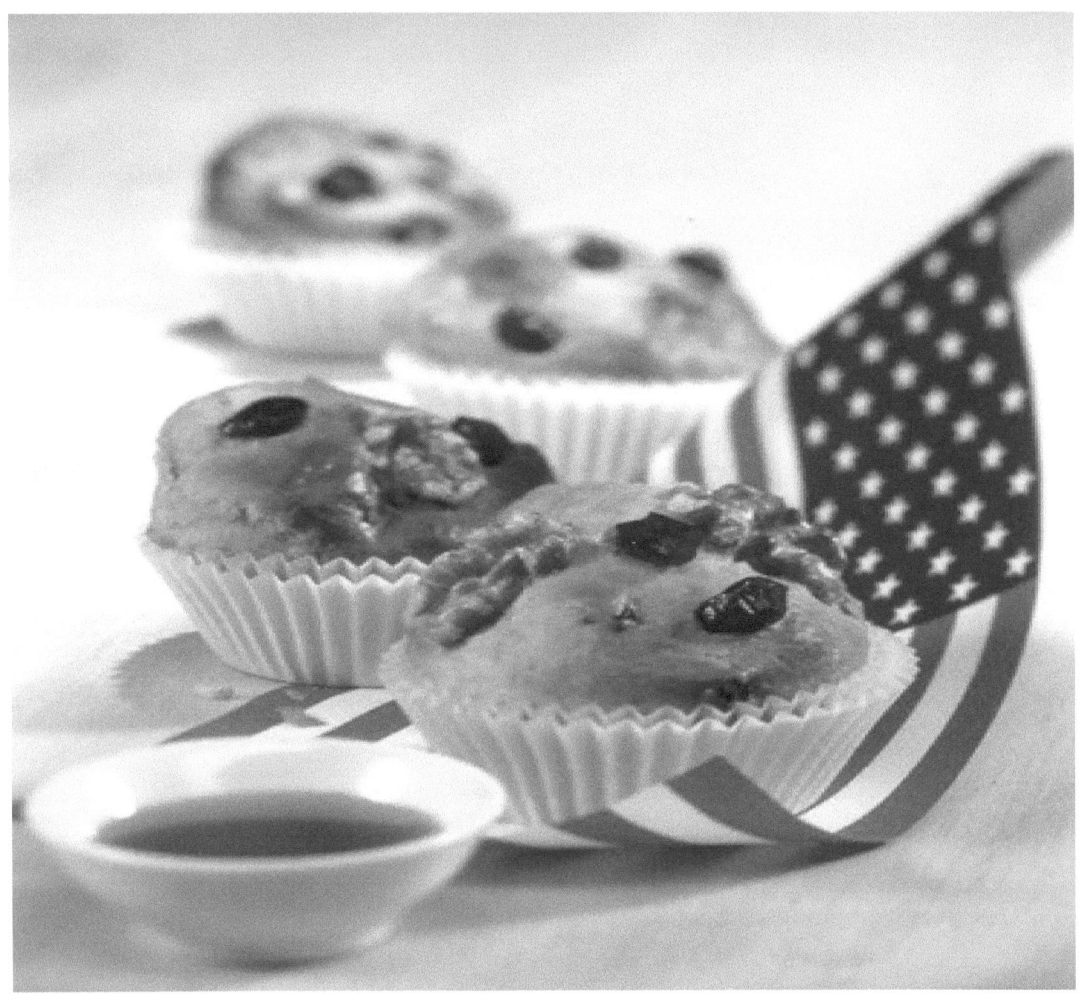

Chocolate nut fruit bars

8 oz couverture (bitter) finely cut the chocolate and melt over a bath of hot water stirring constantly; mix

3-4 tbsp cranberries
3-4 tbsp raisins
2 tbsp pine nuts and
3-4 hazelnuts

into the chocolate lightly oil a flat, rectangular shaped form; coat with cooking foil; spread the chocolate mass evenly; put it in the fridge to set; cut into even-sized pieces

Vanilla and cranberry waffles

Ingredients for about 16 wafers: Mix
1 cup agave sirup or ½ tsp liquid stevia
2 tsp vanilla sugar and
8 oz flour whole grain) stir in
8 or curd
4 eggs and add

8 oz soft butter	with a stirring device to a smooth dough
3 oz cranberries	dried; fold in dough; preheat the waffle iron; pour

dough with a small ladle into the back of the waffle iron; close the lid and bake a few min.

2 tbsp cranberry	fresh, frozen or dried; steam in 1 tsp of butter;

spread powder sugar over the finished waffles and serve with whipped cream

Tip: The fresh hot waffles taste best. They can also be re-baked in the oven immediately before serving at 200 degrees Celsius

Happy Hour: vital food dips & spreads

Chickpea and cranberry puree

1 cup chickpeas	soak overnight; cook in a pot with 3 cups of water for 25 min.; puree with
2 oz cranberries	fresh or frozen; alternate 1-2 tsp powder; puree
3 tbsp sesame oil	
1 tbsp tomato paste	and
¼ tsp of cumin	peel
2 cloves of garlic	finely chop; season with
salt & cayenne	finely chop
½ bn parsley	stir into the puree

Herbal cranberry spread

5 oz organic low-fat quark
5 oz skimmed milk yogurt
2 tbsp of seed or nut oil
1½ oz cranberry, dried	chop; fold in with
4 tbsp of chopped herbs	season with
herbal salt & cayenne	roast
1 tbsp chopped almond	in a frying pan without fat allow

to cool and mix into the spread

Immuno power paste

8 oz low-fat quark	into a bowl mix with
5 tbsp of linseed oil	
3 tbsp linseed	
2 tbsp cranberries	
3 tbsp fresh herb	washed, drained, finely cut, a thumb-thick

2 in piece of ginger peel, finely dice
1 tsp herbal salt,
1 pinch cayenne
1 tsp turmeric	and

2 tbsp liquid seasoning

Tip: This oil-protein-diet based on Johanna Budwig's diet can be changed to suit one's personal taste with curry or chili. If you are often suffering from inflammation, you can always add turmeric to the paste. This spice works just as well as cortisone. If you do not like this plant of the ginger family, you can take 2 capsules a day or wrap turmeric in a rice leaf and swallow the spice with it. If I suffer from inflammation, I give 1 tsp of turmeric and 1 tsp of organic vegetable broth powder into 1 glass of warm water and drink this drink two to three times daily. It is best to use this healthy paste regularly to prevent inflammation

Tofu deli paste

8 oz soft tofu	stir with
5 oz organic soy milk	(unsweetened) and
2 tbsp seed or nut oil	
2 tbsp tomato paste	and

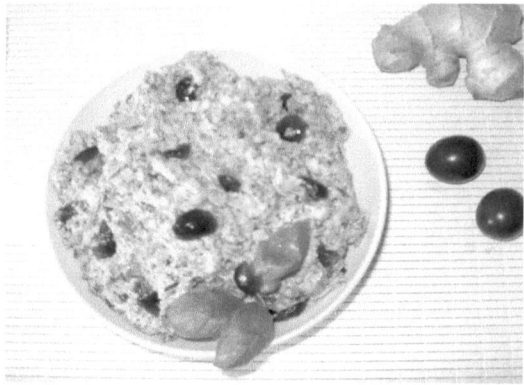

1 tbsp cranberry powder until smooth
1 green onion cut into fine rings
cut 10 filled olives in slices and mix them into the paste; season with
sea salt & cayenne and
2-3 drops stevia

Tart lemon mousse

8 oz soft tofu puree with
½ cup cranberries fresh or frozen and
3 tbsp lemon juice (organic) in a blender; add
2 tbsp almond butter sweeten with
½ tsp stevia

Cranberry mixtures

Anti-stress shake

1 avocado puree the flesh; add
1 tsp cranberry powder and some
chives and stir in
6 oz yogurt season with
salt & cayenne perhaps dilute with water

Artery power drink

10 peeled almonds mix with
½ tsp apple pectin
1 glass cold green tea and
2 oz cranberry sirup or
1 tsp cranberry powder in a blender
sweeten with
2-3 drops stevia

Cashew cranberry mix

¼ cup cashew nuts puree with
¼ cup cranberries fresh or frozen, and
6 oz rice milk in a blender; sweeten with
3-4 drops stevia serve in a champagne coupe; garnish with a mint sprig

Fruity cranberry fizz

2 oz cranberry sirup mix with
2 oz black currant sirup and
¼ tsp soda in a glass of water; if desired sweeten with
some stevia or licorice powder

Cranberry milk liquefy

3 tbsp creamy coconut milk (unsweetened)
1 cup cold rice milk
1½ sup cranberry juice in a blender with
3-4 ice cubes and
1 tsp licorice powder mix into a long drink glass on ice cubes; place a fruit pin with any fruit over the glass rim

Fruity cranberry fizz

½ cup cranberry juice shake with
2 tbsp lemon juice
2 tbsp celery sirup and
2 tbsp grenadine sirup in shaker; fill into a long drink glass on ice cubes; finish with ½ cup of soda water (¼ teaspoon of soda)

Nerve cooler

5 oz oat milk mix with
½ cup cranberry juice
1 tbsp nut butter
1 tbsp chestnut powder sweeten with
3-4 drops stevia garnish with a mint sprig

Paradise punch

¾ cup cranberry juice mix with
2 tbsp almond sirup
4 tbsp orange juice
4 tbsp grapefruit juice add
3-4 ice cubes shake well; pour into a long drink glass

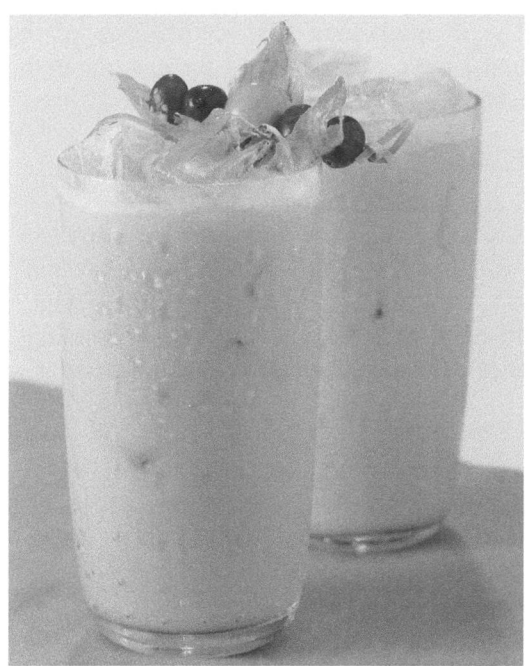

Pineapple cranberry juice

½ organic pineapple — mix with
3-4 oz cranberries — fresh or frozen in a blender

Alternative for those in a hurry: put

1 tsp cranberry powder or 1 capsule into a long drink glass; add
1 can pineapple juice — stir; sweeten with
3- drops stevia

Sweet comforter

6 oz rice milk — mix with
½ cup cranberries — fresh or frozen
1/3 cup mint leaves
1-2 tbsp walnuts — and
5 drops stevia — or 1 tsp. licorice powder in a blender; decorate with a mint sprig

Thanksgiving punch

1 ginger root — thumb-sized; peel; cut in thin slices; with
1 tbsp mulled wine spice or
1 stick of cinnamon
2 cloves
1 pinch cardamom — and
1 pinch pimento — in a tea ball
16 oz cranberry juice
16 z orange juice — and
2 tbsp agave sirup — alternatively sugar or ½ teaspoon stevia;
bring to a boil, remove from the heat and allow soaking for 10 minutes
4 kumquats — wash cut into slices
2 tbsp cranberries — (fresh) toss them in sugar and attach them on
the edge of the punch glasses; pour the hot cranberry punch into prepared glasses.

In each glass, add some kumquat slices and cinnamon sticks to stir. Tip: Ice-cooled, garnished with fresh mint leaves, the cranberry

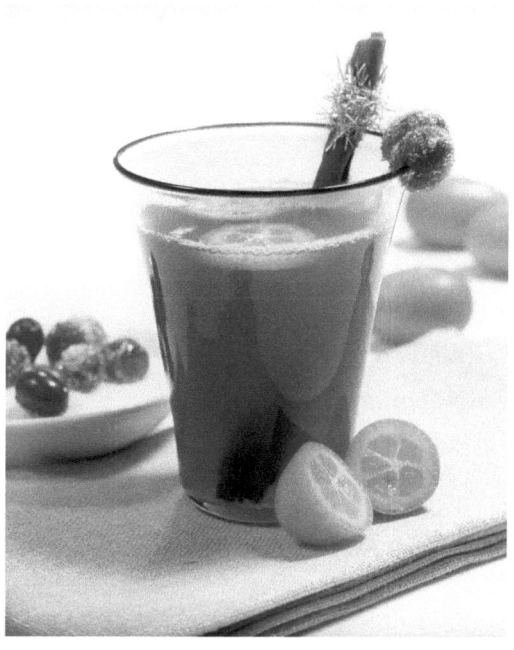

punch is an excellent aperitif for summer festivals. Kumquats have been cultivated in China for 4000 years, but now also in Israel, Italy, and Japan. The citrus fruits look like tiny oval oranges. The fruit is sweet-sour, the edible shell somewhat bitter. If you roll them slightly between your fingers before eating, they become softer and sweeter. A friend breeds the trees himself and eats 2-3 Kumquats daily to clean his blood. In this way, he has lived with a leukemia species for more than 20 years.

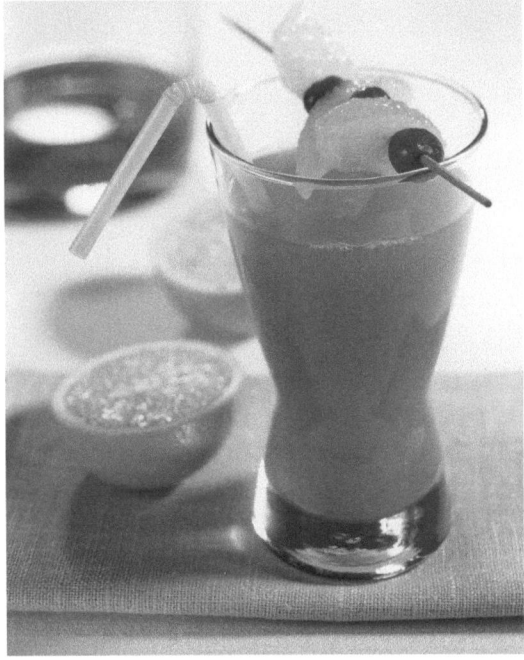

Cocktails & Dreams

Cosmopolitan   put

2 cl vodka lemon
4 cl cranberry juice
1 cl Cointreau and
1 cl of lime juice   in a shaker; add 3 to 4 ice cubes and shake vigorously

The Cosmopolitan has become one of the best-known cocktails since the mention in the television series Sex and the City

Pink Dream

2 cl cranberry sirup   mix with
8 cl orange juice   and some ice cubes in a long drink glass with a bar spoon; fill up with
10 cl of bitter lemon; decorate with orange slices, fresh cranberries or cocktail cherries

Cran-Apple

3 oz of cranberry juice,
3 oz apple wine and
¼ tsp of soda   with some ice water

Cranberry Collins   stir

2 cl vodka
1 cl elderflower cordial
2 cl cranberry sirup   and
some ice cubes   with a bar spoon and fill up with soda

Sex on the Beach   shake

2 tbsp peach liqueur
2 tbsp vodka
½ cup cranberry juice or 1 capsule powder
½ cup pineapple juice with ice in the shaker; serve the cocktail in a long drink glass

Save Sex on the Beach

For 2-4 persons
9 fl oz pinaepple juice with
9 fl oz cranberry juice and
2 tbsp coconut milk   (unsweetened, creamy) Shake with ice and serve in champagne glasses; add
1 tsp coconut cream   and garnish with mint leaves

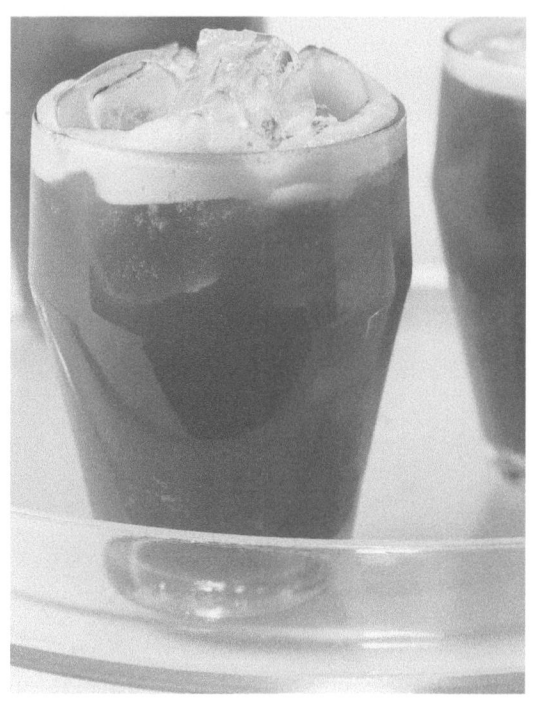
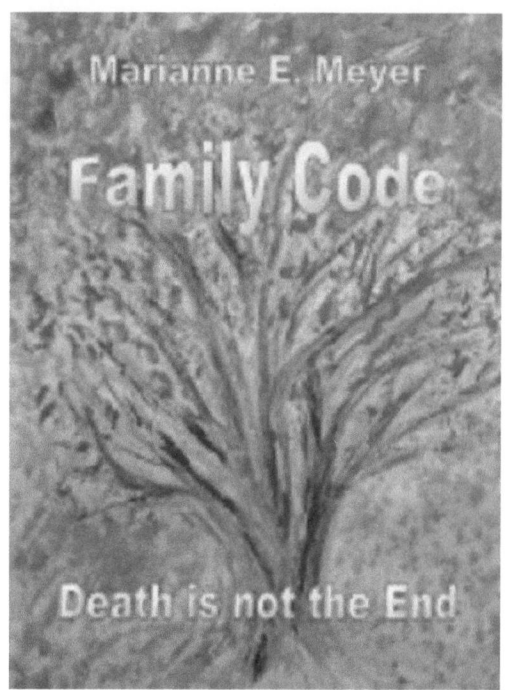

Cranberry Colada

½ cup Pina Colada   Mix
1 cup ice cubes   and
1 tbsp of cranberry juice in blender;
fill the cocktail glasses and garnish with ice and fresh cranberries

Vocal cord delight

½ cup oat milk   mix with
2 tbsp lemon juice
2 tbsp advocaat   and
2 tbsp cranberry sirup

During the rehearsal of our Gospel choir with the drum group Bingoma

Https://www.youtube.com/watch?v=RDOdzkf6EOc

I'd created this drink because egg liqueur or raw egg yolk is known to oil stressed vocal cords; by sipping it hoarseness will vanish

In this captivating spiritual novel takes the reader part in Marianne's exciting life on four continents. Her experiences clarify that we are all interconnected and for generations, families have their value system. This code of rules, sayings and communication styles is also reflected when the family members do not know each other or are living on different continents.

ISBN:978-3741282331   184 p. 17x22cm €8,98

Free forum for free questions

Dear reader! Perhaps you have already had to deal with one or more health problems mentioned in the book and might have already found a solution or have been much more involved. If you would like to share it, you can send me an email to

drmarianneemeyer @ gmail.com

Or leave a comment on one of my blogs about CRANBERRY on my website. Then it would be possible for all readers consulting my domain to benefit from your experience:

www.marianne-e-meyer.de

In the end, all that remains to be desired is to wish you all the best on your way to the light, to inner freedom, to serenity, and to radiant health! Thank you for your trust!

Acknowledgments

Finally, I would like to thank you very sincerely for all those spiritual and physical helpers who were involved in the book:

I am particularly close to the Russian doctor, Alfira Weihe, who lives in Bielefeld. She contacted me at the right moment. Without her question, if she could translate my Spirulabuch, the boss of the Windpferd publishing house Monika Jünemann would have made the Cranberry hardly palatable.

I would like to thank some of the friends from near and far for the many proofs of the existence of morphogenic fields:

Carole Madrid, Leanne Dodge, Betty Roehm, Ursula Keim, Renée Stellwag, and Elisabeth Fleischer.

Since I could only find very little material about the large-fruited cranberry in the Anglo-American area, I'm grateful to the medical practitioner Michael Gracher and Anja Binger of the company GSE for literature and an extra portion of cranberry powder. In the brochure of the CMC Cranberry Marketing Committee "Die Kraftbeere", Technical Information for the Food Industry, "I came across the Bonn marketing and communications company mk2 gmbh: I thank Maria Kraus, Kristina Moss, Inga Klein and Sam Bessinger for their friendly service.

My thanks also go to Jennifer Christoph from the Cranberry Information Center in Frankfurt, Dr. Renate Kaiser-Alexnat, Bob Hartmann, Edith Holschuh, Claudia Trossmann, Hilde Richter-Hudson and Ursula Keim for literature, information, and tips. Also to all, who gave me by experience reports or advice and act but here not mentioned by name very heartfelt thanks!

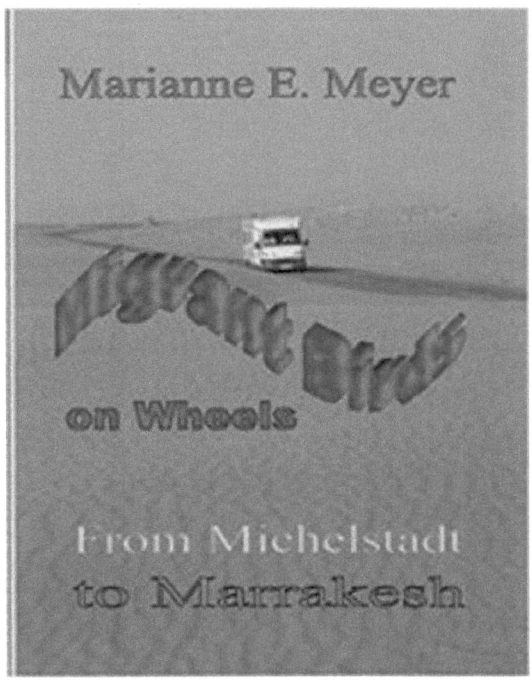

If your attention span is suffering from this reading matter, I can offer you this exciting book. In this novel form, health tips come from medical miracles on two legs that we have met in Morocco. But do not expect a guide. The book is something for Morocco insiders.

REFERENCES

Amieva, Peek RM jr: Pathobiology of Helicobacter pylori-Induced Gastric Cancer. Gastroenterology. 2016 Jan;150(1):64-78

Anhê, FF et al.: A polyphenol-rich cranberry extract protects from diet-induced obesity, insulin resistance and intestinal inflammation in association with increased Akkermansia spp. Population in the gut microbiota of mice. Gut. 2015 Jun;64(6):872-83.

Avorn J et al.:Reduction of bacteriuria and pyuria after ingestion of cranberry juice. JAMA1994 Mar 9;271(10):751-4.

Bone, RA et al.: Lutein and zeaxanthin in the eyes, serum and diet of human subjects. Exp Eye Res 2000; 71(3) 239-45

Bone, RA et al.: Macular pigment in donor eyes with and without AMD: a case-control study. Invest. Ophthalmal. Vis Sci. 2001; 42: 235-40

Boon, PC et al.: Effects of Lutein from Marigold Extract on Immunity and Growth of Mammary Tumors in Mice. Anticancer Research 1996; 16:3689-94

Burger, O.et al.: Inhibition of Helicobacter pylori adhesion to human gastric mucus by a high-molecular-weight constituent of cranberry juice. Crit Rev Food Sci Nutr. 2002; 42(3 Suppl):279-84

Cavanagh, H.M. Hipwell, M. und Wilkinson: Antibacterial activity of berry fruits used for culinary purposes. J Med Food. 2003 Spring; 6(1): 57-61

Chambers, BK, Camire, M.E.: Can Cranberry Supplementation Benefit Adults With Type 2 Diabetes? *Diabetes Care* 26:2695-2696, 2003

Chang CH et al.: Photoprotective effects of cranberry juice and its various fractions against blue light-induced impairment in human retinal pigment epithelial cells. Pharm Biol. 2017 Dec; 55 (1):571-580

Carabin IG, FlammWG: Evaluation of safety of inulin and oligofructose as dietary fiber. Regul Toxicol Pharmacol.1999 Dec;30(3):268-82.

Cipollini, ML, Stiles, EW: Antifungal activity of ripe ericaceous fruits: phenolic-acid interactions and palatability for dispersers. Biochem Syst Ecol 1992;20:501-14

Dagnelie, G et al.: Lutein improves visual function in some patients with retinal degeneration: a pilot study via the Internet. Optometry 2000, Mar; 71(3):147-64.

Ferguson, PJ et al: A flavonoid fraction from cranberry extract inhibits proliferation of human tumor cell lines. J Nutr. 2004 Jun; 134(6):1529-35

Frasetto L, Kohlstadt I: Treatment and prevention of kidney stones: an update. Am Fam Physician, 2011 Dec 1;84(11):1234-42

Girardot, M et al.: Promising results of cranberry in the prevention of oral Candida biofilms. Pathog Dis. 2014 Apr;70(3):432-9

Grant, P : Warfarin and cranberry juice: an interaction? J Heart Valve Dis. 2004 Jan;13(1):25-6

Greenberg, JA., Newman, S.J., Howell, A.B.: Consumption of sweetened dried cranberries versus unsweetened raisins for inhibition of uropathogenic Escherichia coli adhesion in human urine: a pilot study. J Altern Complement Med. 2005 Oct; 11(5):875-8

Han, TL et al.:The metabolic basis of Candida albicans morphogenesis and quorum sensing. Fungal Genet Biol. 2011 Aug;48(8):747-63

Heaton, S: Organic farming, food quality and human health: A review of the evidence. Soil Association, Bristol 2001

Howell AB, Vorsa N, Marderosian AD, Foo LY. Inhibition of the adherence of p-fimbriated Escherichia coli to uroepithelial-cell surfaces by proanthocyanidin extracts from cranberries. New England Journal of Medicine 1998; 339:1085.

Howell AB, Leahy M, Kurowska E, Guthrie N. In vivo evidence that cranberry proanthocyanidins inhibit adherence of p-fimbriated E. coli bacteria to uroepithelial cells. Federation of American Societies for Experimental Biology Journal 2001; 15:A284.

Howell, AB, Foxman, B.: Cranberry juice and adhesion of antibiotic-resistant uropathogens. JAMA. 2002 Jun 19; 287(23):3082-3

Jiadong S et al.: Cranberry (Vaccinium macrocarpon) oligosaccharides decrease biofilm formation by uropathogenic Escherichia coli. Journal of Functional Foods. Volume 17, August 2015, Pages 235–242

Kreutz, G et al.: Effects of choir singing or listening on secretory immunoglobulin A, cortisol, and emotional state. J Behav Med, 2004 Dec; 27(6):623-35

Kruse-Elliott, K et al.: Paper presentation: Cranberry juice modulates atherosclerotic vascular dysfunction, April 3, Physiology 387.14/board #A661. 35th Congress of the International Union of Physiological Sciences in San Diego, March 31 - April 5, 2005.

Kongress der Internationalen Vereinigung für Physiologie in San Diego, vom 31. März bis 5. April 2005

Kontiokari T, Sundqvist K, Nuutinen M, Pokka T, Koskela M, Uhari M. Randomised trial of cranberry-lingonberry juice and Lactobacillus GG drink for the prevention of urinary tract infections in women. British Medical Journal 2001; 322:1571-1575.

Kontiokari T, Laitinen J, Jarvi L, Pokka T, Sundqvist K, Uhari M. Dietary factors protecting women from urinary tract infection. American Journal of Clinical Nutrition 2003; 77:600-604.

Küster, Ernst: Lehrbuch der Botanik für Mediziner. Leipzig, 1920

Ledda A et al.: Highly standardized cranberry extract supplementation (Anthocran®) as prophylaxis in young healthy subjects with recurrent urinary tract infections. EurRevMed Pharmacol Sci. 2017 Jan;21(2):389-393

Matsushima, M et al.: Growth inhibitory action of cranberry on Helicobacter pylori. Gastroenertologie. doi:10.1111/j.1440-1746.2008.05409

Meyer, Marianne E: Spirulina, das blaugrüne Wunder, 7. Auflage, Aitrang 2006
Family Code, Norderstedt 2017

Neumann, Halima: Stop Azidose, Allergie und Haarausfall, Starnberg 1994

Nothlings, U, Kolonel, LN: Risk factors for pancreatic cancer in the Hawaii-Los Angeles Multiethnic Cohort Study. Hawaii Med J. 2006 Jan; 65(1): 26-8

Ofek I, Goldhar J, Zafriri D, Lis H., Adar R, Sharon N.: Anti-Escherichia coli adhesion activity of cranberry and blueberry juices. New England Journal of Medicine 1991; 324:1599

Parry. J et al: Chemical compositions, antioxidant capacities, and antiproliferative activities of selected fruit seed flours.J Agric Food Chem. 2006 May 31;54(11):3773-8

Puupponen-Pimia R et al.: The action of berry phenolics against human intestinal pathogens. 1: Biofactors, 2005; 23(4):243-51

Rindone, JP,Murphy, TW*American Journal of Therapeutics.* Warfarin-Cranberry Juice, Interaction Resulting in Profound Hypoprothrombinemia and Bleeding. 13(3):283-284, May/June 2006

Rolfs, A et al.: Prevalence of Fabry disease in patients with cryptogenic stroke: a prospective study. Lancet. 2005 Nov 19; 366(9499):1754-6 urgesund", 7. Aufl . 2005

Sobota AE: Inhibition of bacterial adherence by cranberry juice: potential use for the treatment of urinary tract infections. Journal of Urology 1984; 131:1013-1016

Stothers, L: A randomized trial to evaluate effectiveness and cost effectiveness of naturopathic cranberry products as prophylaxis against urinary tract infection in women. Can J Urol. 2002 Jun; 9(3):1558-62.

Sun, J, Cu, YF, Wu, X, Liu, RH: Antioxidant and antiproliferative activities of common fruits. J Agric Food Chem.2002, Dec 4; 50(25): 7449-54

Sun, J, Hai Liu, R: Cranberry phytochemical extract induce cell arrest an apoptosis in human MCF-7 breast cancer cells. Cancer Lett. 2005 Dec 22

Swartz, JH, Medrek TF: Antifungal properties of cranberry juice. Appl Microbiol 1968; 16: 1524-7.

Trainer Thompson, Jennifer: Very Cranberry, Berkeley 2003

Walker EB, Barney DP, Mickerlsen JN, Walton RJ, Mickelsen RAJr. Cranberry concentrate: UTI prophylaxis. Journal of Family Practice 1997; 45:167-168.

Weh, KM, Clarke, J, Kresty, LA: Cranberries and

Cancer: An Update of Preclinical Studies Evaluating the Cancer Inhibitory Potential of Cranberry and Cranberry Derived Constituents. Antioxidants (Basel) 2016 Aug 18;5(3).

Weiss, EI et al: Inhibiting interspecies coaggregation of plaque bacteria with a cranberry juice constituent. Journal of the American Dental Association 1998; 129:1719-1723.

Weiss, EI: A high molecular mass cranberry constituent reduces mutans streptococci level in saliva and inhibits in vitro adhesion to hydroxyapatite. J Americ Dent. Assoc. TEMS Microb. Letters, March 2004 (232): 89

Widmer, Regina: Praxiserfahrung zum postkoitalen Urethralsyndrom. Harnröhre, Blase und das Intimleben der Frau. In: Schweizer Zeitschrift für Gynäkologie und Geburtshilfe in der Praxis, 5/05.

Zhang L, Ma J, Pan K, Go V, Chen J, You W. Efficacy of Cranberry Juice on Helicobacter pylori Infection: a Double-Blind, Randomized Placebo-Controlled Trial. Helicobacter 2005; 10:139-145.

Zhu, M et al.: Effects of long-term cranberry supplementation on endocrine pancreas in aging rats. J Gerontol A Biol Sci Med Sci. 2011 Nov; 66(11):1139-51

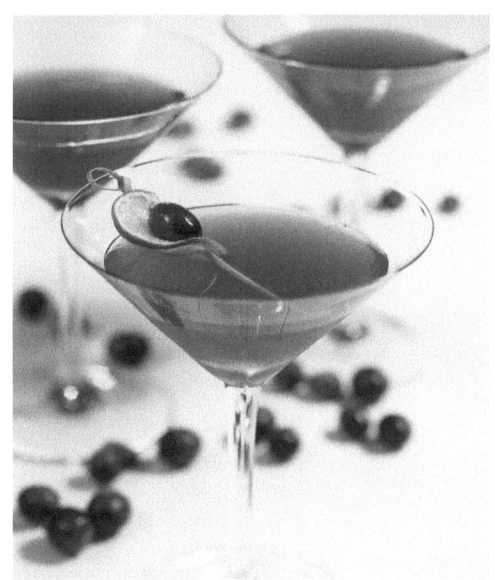

Alphabetic index

Acidic food 11,32,40,44,46
Acupressure 44
Acupuncture 44
Agave sirup 14,17,18,76,80,83
Agitation 13
Alcohol 13-15,41,43,52
Algae 10,36,42
Alkaline 33,36,52,57,95
Almonds 17,26,58,69,77,82
    milk 58
Aloe vera 42,50
Aloe vera essence 50
Alpha-linolenic acid 35
Alpha lipoic acid 39
AMD 31,44,45,47,50,51
Amylase 46
Anesthetics 36
Anti-adhesion effect 47,50,51
Antibiotics 13,14,20,35,44
Anti-candida diet 11,14,36
Anticoagulant 48,49
Antioxidants 11,15,28,29,31-33,38,39,41,47,
    52,56
Antiviral 27
Anthocran® 34
Apple cider 39
Apple pectin 74,76,78,79,82
Arbutin 27,51
Arteriosclerosis 28,33,48,52
Acetylsalicylic acid (ASA) or Aspirin® 48
Arthritis 37,46,48,95
Asparagus 14
    salad 60
Aspartame 17
Autoimmune diseases 46,48
Autonomous nervous system 42
Avocados 14,38,63,82
Bactericidal 27
Bacteriuria 49
Bananas 13,14,26,30,41
Barley grass (juice) 14,50

Bearberry leaf 51
Bear leek 33
Beta carotene 31,32,44
Bilberry (*Vaccinium uliginosum*) 19,27,39
Bile 37,75
Biliary salts 46
Biofeedback 44
Biofilm 51
Birch 51
Bitter melon 39
Blackberry 35
Black radish 57
Bladder 13-16,20,26-28,34,37,40,43,44,50-57
   cancer 28,
   irritable 10,43,44
   infection 13,20,27,34,37,52,54,55
   pain 17
   tea 20
Bleeding gums 45
Blood-brain barrier 31
Blood coagulation inhibitors 48
Blood glucose level 29,37,38
Blood vessels 17,29,33,4047
Blue agave 14
Blueberry 29
Blue light 31
Brain attacks 47
Brain cancer 35
Breathing exercises 52
Breast cancer 35
Broccoli 37
Buckhorn 34
Buckwheat 33,57
Budwig, Johanna 40,81
Burning sensation 13,14,29,34,37,43,51
Buttermilk 73
Cabbage juice 34
Calcium phosphate stones 44
Cancer 15,16,26,28,29,32,34,35,39,56,76
Candida (yeast overgrowth) 13,14,35,36,
                40,41,45,56
Capillaries 30

Carbohydrates 19,31
Cardiac insufficiency 13
Cardiovascular diseases 33,40,45,47,48
Caries 20,26,32,36,40,45,46
Carotenoids 28,31,44,69
Catalase 39
Cataract 31,36,37
Carrots 57,61,69,72,73
Cayce, Edgar 49
Cayenne pepper 39,58,60-65,67,69,70,72-75
                81,82
Celery 46,50,70,71,73,82
Cerebral hemorrhage 47
Cerebral vein 41
Chamomile 40
Chardonnay grape 35
Chestnuts 57
Chia seeds 58,73
Chicory 14,60
Chlorella 37
Chocolate 27,30,47,50,77,79,80
Cholesterol 19,29,30,33,40,41,47
Chronic renal disease 44
Cilantro 37,62,65
Cinnamon 39,77,83
Circulatory diseases 11,28,32,33,41
Clove /oil 40,73,74,83
CMC Cranberry Marketing Committee 30
Coconut oil/creme 58,69-72
Coffee 33,43,52
Cold feet 34,37,43,56
Collagen 30,37
Colloidal gold 36
Colloidal silver 13,14,36,42,46,51
Concentration problems 55
Combustion 29
Copper 31,39
Corn/flour/starch 57,73,74
Coronary capillary 41
Cortisol 42
Cortisone 81
Cottage cheese 40

Cowberry 11,15,20,26,27
Cow's milk 37,56,60
Cranberry (*Vaccinium macrocarpon*)
   chocolate 47,77
   concentrate 17-19,39
   Early Black 21
   flavored 19,50
   frozen 19,69,76,78,81-83
   highbush (*Viburnum opulus*) 26
   jelly 11,24,77
   juice 13-21,24-27,30,31,34-57,69,74,78, 82
   ice cubes 57,82,85,85
   light juice 41
   Mc Farlin 21
   mouthwash 16,36,46
   Paradise Meadow
   powder 16-19,24,26,31,33,35,38,39,41, 45,48,52,55-58,6277,82-84,86
   sirup 17,19,41,45,46,51,5377,78,82,84,85
   sweetened 18,19
Curd 40,66,67,80
Cystitis 13,14,34,37,51
Dental plaque 45
Detoxifying plants 37
Diabetes 13,37,38,40,45,95
Diuretics 44
DNA 29,30,41
Drugs 13,32,35,36,44,45
Dulcamara 44
Edema 30
Energy 26,29,31,36,41,52,55,56,95
Enterobacteriaceae 46
Enzymes 36-39,46
Escherichia coli bacteria 16,34
Eyes/inflamed/ lens 36,37,44,45,57
Fat 17,19,29,31-33,35,46,47,57
Fatty acids, saturated 32
Fatty acids, monounsaturated 32
Fatty acids, polyunsaturated 32
Fiber 19,22,28,31,37,49
Field horsetail 33

Figs 41,57
Flavonoids 28,33
Floss 45
Folate 32
Food poisoning 39,47
FOS (fructooligosaccharides) 14,78
Free radicals 29,39,44
Frequent urination 14,34,37
Fungi 13,14,23,27,*28*,35,36,40,45,56
Fungicidal 27
Fusel alcohols 41
Garlic 14,40,48,60-62,65,69,72-74,81
Gastric cancer/juices/ ulcers 16,39,40,46,47
Gastrointestinal viruses 42
Geum alpina 39
Ginger 18,20,40,58,65,70,81,83
Gingival fibroblasts 40
Gingival pocket 40
Gingivitis 40,45,46
Ginkgo 18
Glioblastoma 28
Glutathione peroxidase 39
Glycerine 19
Glycolytic process 36
Golden potentila aurea 39
Goldenrod 34,51
Gout 46
Grapefruit seed extract 13,14,36,51
Green tea 36,40,50,82
Gums/disease/inflammation 20,28,32,40,45
Harvest 21-24
   dry 24
   wet 24
HDL (*good*) cholesterol 41
Healing clay 40
Heart disease 17,28,33,34,40,41
Heart attack 33,41,47
Heather plant 27
Helicobacter pylori bacteria 16,39
High blood pressure 30,47
Hippuric acid 27
Hoodia 10

Homosporous plants 15
Horseradish 58,60,67
Horsetail 51
Hydrochloric acid 46
Hydrogen peroxide (H2O2) 51
Hydroquinone 51
Hydroxyl radicals 30
Hyperactivity 17
Hypochondriacs 48
Hypothrombinemia 48
Ibuprofen 48
Immune defense 2,45
Immune deficiency 41
Immune system 10,11,14,26,28-32,36,41,42, 55,56
Immunoglobulin A 42,45
Inflammation 13,17,30,34,35,37-40,42,45,49, 51,57,81
Interleukin-6 40
Intestinal flora 14,35
Intestinal infections 42
Intestine 14,16,36,37,41,42,46
Intimate sprays 37
Ionizing radiation 32
Irritable bladder 10,43,44
Iron 19,27,31,39
Juniper 51
Karach, Fedor 36
Kefir 14
Kidney 20,34,35,37,42,47,50,51,57
Kidney stones 37,44
    calcium phosphate 44
    struvite 44
Kumquats 83,84
Künzle, Johann 39
Lactobacilli 36
Lady's mantle tea 44
Lapacho tea 36
Laughing 41
LDL (*bad*) cholesterol 29,30,47
Legumes 57
Linseed/yellow 40,60

Licorice powder 63,82,83
Linseed oil 40
Lipase 46
Lipids 31,32,41
Lutein 31,32,44
Lymphoma 2
Itching 13
Jícama leeks 14
Lemons 44,58
Leukemia 34
Lingonberry 15,26
Low urine volume 34,37
Macular degeneration 31,44
Magnesium 17,31,40
Manganese 39
Marcumar 48
Marigold 42
Matrix metalloproteinase-3 40
Macula lutea 44
Meat 11,24,26,34,39,46,47,58,69
Methuselahs 52,53
Microbes 39,51
Microbiome 14
Micturition diary 43
Migraine 17
Millet 57
Minerals 28,31,36,40
Mistletoe 33
Monosodium glutamate 17
Moors 15,24
Mucous congestion 37
Multiplasan mineral complex 33,36
Muscle cramps 43
Mustard 58
Mycosis 35
Myocardial infarction 47
Nearsightedness 30
Nephrolithiasis 44
Nerve supply, lack of 37
Nettle 51
Nicotine 43
Nocturia 13

Nutmeg 39,75
Ocean Spray 41
Oligomeric procyanidins (OPC) 29-31,36,37, 47
Olives 36,57,62,82
Omega-3 fatty acids 33
Organic products 17
Osteoporosis 17,37
Overactive bladder 43
Overmanning 34
Oxygen 44
Pain 13,15,46,49,54,55,90
Painkillers 30
Pancreas 37
Pancreatic cancer 34
Pancreatitis 44
Papaya 14,36,38
Parasites 13,41,45
Pepsin 46
Periodontal disease 36,40
Periodontitis 40
Plaques 11,29,33
Phenols 40
Phosphorus 31
Phytochemicals 26
Pineapple 17,51,76
Plaque bacteria 36
Platelets 47
Plum 29
Poor digestion 46
Polyarthritis 46
Polyphenols 28,29
polyunsaturated fatty acids
Postmenopausal estrogen deficiency 37
Postoperative hemorrhages 48
Potassium 31,40
Potatoes 13,57
Prevention 29,32-34,36,44,45,48,50,51
Proanthocyanidins (PAC) 16,29,49,50
Probiotics 14,35,78
Prostate cancer 35
Protease inhibitors 44

Protein 19,28,29,31,37,40,41,49,65
Proteus mirabilis microbes 46
Prothrombin 48
Provitamin A (retinol) 31
Psyllium husks 2,58
Pubis pain 37
Pulsatilla 44
Pumpkin 37
Pumpkin seeds 51
Pyuria 49
Quinic acid 27
Radical scavengers 38
Radio waves 32
Red blood cells 42
Red wine 29,41
Renal disease/insufficiency 34,37,51
Restharrow 51
Resveratrol 34
Retina 30,44
retinal pigment epithelium (ARPE-19) 44
Rheumatism 37,42,46
Rheumatoid arthritis 46
Rods 51
Roots 22a 36
Salicylic acid 51
Saliva 36,40,41,45
Salmonella 39,46
Salmonellosis 47
Sauerkraut 14
Sausage 39
Scurvy 15,25
Saweed preparations 54
Secondary plant compounds (metabolites) 28 41,
Selenium 31,37
Sesame oil 58
Shigella 46
Shoots 22
Sodium 31,41
Soy flour/sauce 58
Speedwell 33
Spelt 57

Spheres 51
Spices, hot 51
Spirulina
Spores 15
Sprouts 22,28
Staphylococci 37
Stevia 17,44
Stomach acid 39
Stomach cancer 39
Strawberries 29
Streptococcus mutans 36
Stress 15
Stress acids 40
Stroke 33
Struvite stones 44
Sugar 31
Sunflower oil 36
    seeds
Superoxide dismutase (SOD) 39
Swedish herbs 42
Taboulé 61
Tampons 37
Tannins, condensed 27,56
Taurine 39
Tea, black 52
Thrombosis 30,48
Thyme 47
Thyroid 26,54
Tofu 58
Tooth decay 26,36
Topinambour 14
Trypsin 46
Tumeric 40,60
Ulcer 16,42,47
Urethra 34,37
Urethral infection 13
Urge to urinate 13,43,51,53-55
Urine, blood in 37,55
Urinary tract/infection   10,13,16,17,20,26,27,
          29,32,34,35,42-46,48-51,56
Uroepithelial cells 35
UV rays 31

Vaccines 36
Vaccinium macrocarpon 15
Vaccinium vitis-idaea 15
Vegetative nervous system 43
Virus 28,42,45
Vitamins 28,29,31
Vitamin A 29,31
Vitamin B1 (thiamine) 31
Vitamin B2 (riboflavin) 31
Vitamin B3 (niacin)
Vitamin C (ascorbic acid – E 300) 25,3
Vitamin E (alpha-tocopherol) 31
amin E (alpha-tocopherol) mg 1.20
Vitamin K (phylloquinone) 31
Warfarin 48
Water 2,11,17-20,22,24,26,29,31,35,39-42,
        44,47,51,53-57,81,95
Wheat grass juice 50
Whey powder, sweet 57
White beans 57,58

Wild herbs 37
Yarrow 37
Yeast /overgrowth/infection 11,13,14,35, 45,
        54
Yoga 52
Yogurt 13,60
Xanthophyll 31
X-rays 36
Zeaxanthin 31
Zinc 31,37
Zucchini 61

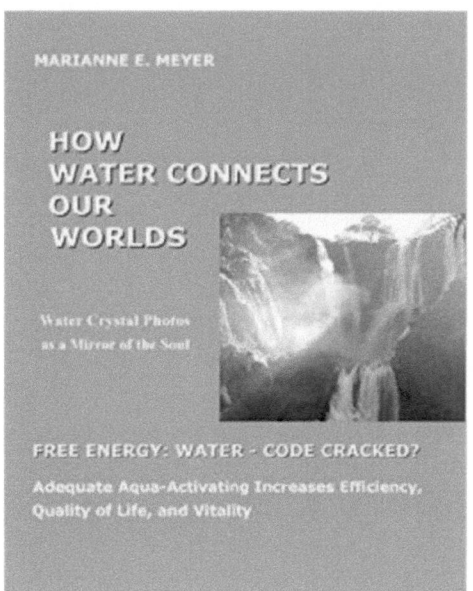 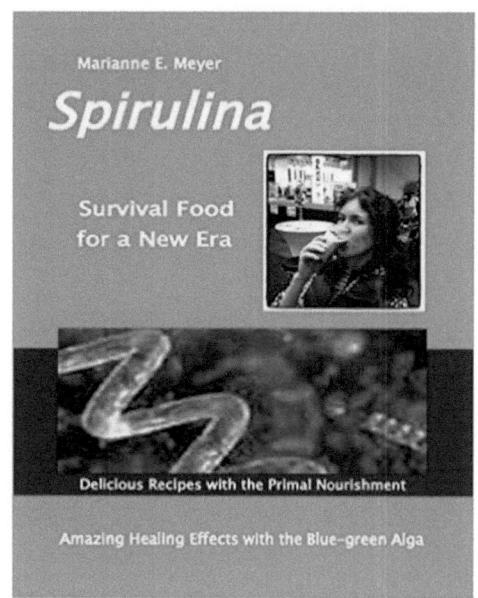

This captivating book wins by a clear statement on the mystery of changeability and storage ability of the water. Inge Schneider, head of the Swiss Jupiter-Verlag, found in her book review in the NET-Journal the author's findings that the water is the "interface between the physical and metaphysical reality" particularly appealing.

The reader will find disturbing facts about the quality of commercial waters. Anyone who believes that a tap water is clean, is encouraged to think and act. M. Meyer advises to activating water adequately. After all, who tastes for the first time naturally vitalized, oxygenated and alkaline water from the tap, want to drink no more soda water from plastic bottles. Pure water is the ideal solution for all health problems, especially if they affect the brain.

Ultimately, the author introduces free energy researchers and their technologies. She also shows what to do, so space energy can soon flow in all households.

ISBN 978-3734736919 104 p. 17x22cm €7,99

We all need Spirulina. Why? Because of infertile soils, we can hardly get energy from our food. The blue-green alga is concentrated solar power since it contains all the colors of the spectrum and thus all frequencies of light, just like the water of Lourdes.

Marianne Erika Meyer introduced Spirulina, the blue-green miracle via her same-named German bestseller and an appearance on Prime TV in German-speaking Europe and Russia. Ever more people supplement their diets with the beneficial protein food. And dentists use it progressively for discharging amalgam and other poisons.

Stunning studies & reports around the globe prove: With Spirulina we strengthen our immune system as well as stand up to pain, depression, diabetes, MS, cataracts, allergies, anemia, arthritis, liver fibrosis, Parkinson's disease, and even AIDS and cancer.

In the illustrated book with delicious recipes, the doctor of nutrition covered each chapter in note form and highlighted important parts.

ISBN 978-3734728525 104 p. 17x22cm €7,99

FOR YOUR NOTES

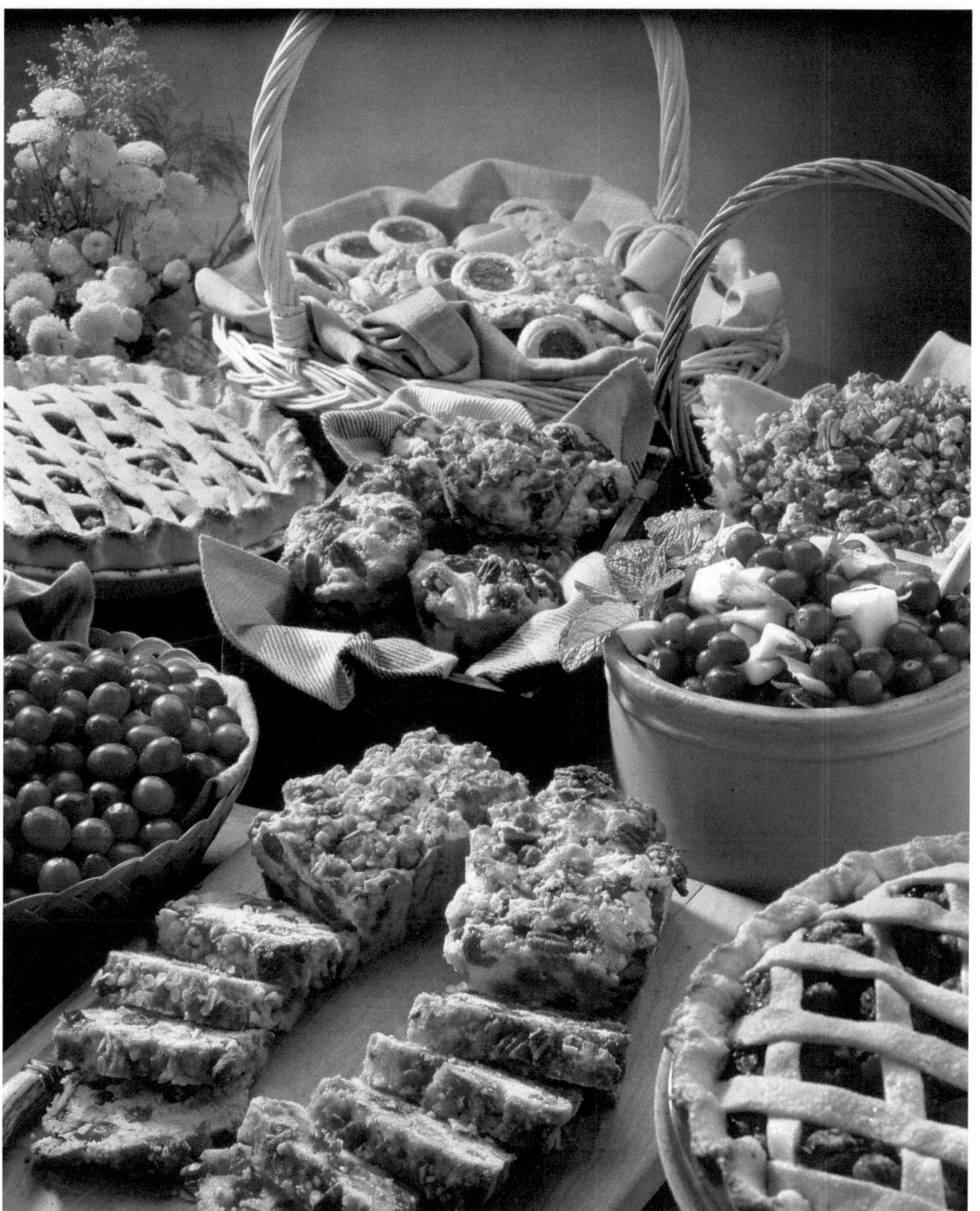

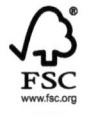